W9-BKL-040

Nursing Leadership and Management
Review Module Edition 6.0

CONTRIBUTORS

Sheryl Sommer, PhD, RN, CNE
VP Nursing Education & Strategy

Janean Johnson, MSN, RN
Nursing Education Strategist

Karin Roberts, PhD, MSN, RN, CNE
Nursing Education Coordinator

Sharon R. Redding, EdD, RN, CNE
Nursing Education Specialist and Content Project Coordinator

Lois Churchill, MN, RN
Nursing Education Specialist

EDITORIAL AND PUBLISHING

Derek Prater
Spring Lenox
Michelle Renner
Mandy Tallmadge
Kelly Von Lunen

CONSULTANTS

Linda Turchin, MSN, RN, CNE

Intellectual Property Notice

Important Notice to the Reader

Assessment Technologies Institute, LLC, is the publisher of this publication. The content of this publication is for informational and educational purposes only and may be modified or updated by the publisher at any time. This publication is not providing medical advice and is not intended to be a substitute for professional medical advice, diagnosis, or treatment. The publisher has designed this publication to provide accurate information regarding the subject matter covered; however, the publisher is not responsible for errors, omissions, or for any outcomes related to the use of the contents of this book and makes no guarantee and assumes no responsibility or liability for the use of the products and procedures described or the correctness, sufficiency, or completeness of stated information, opinions, or recommendations. The publisher does not recommend or endorse any specific tests, providers, products, procedures, processes, opinions, or other information that may be mentioned in this publication. Treatments and side effects described in this book may not be applicable to all people; likewise, some people may require a dose or experience a side effect that is not described herein. Drugs and medical devices are discussed that may have limited availability controlled by the Food and Drug Administration (FDA) for use only in a research study or clinical trial. Research, clinical practice, and government regulations often change the accepted standard in this field. When consideration is being given to use of any drug in the clinical setting, the health care provider or reader is responsible for determining FDA status of the drug, reading the package insert, and reviewing prescribing information for the most up-to-date recommendations on dose, precautions, and contraindications and determining the appropriate usage for the product. Any references in this book to procedures to be employed when rendering emergency care to the sick and injured are provided solely as a general guide. Other or additional safety measures may be required under particular circumstances. This book is not intended as a statement of the standards of care required in any particular situation, because circumstances and a patient's physical condition can vary widely from one emergency to another. Nor is it intended that this book shall in any way advise personnel concerning legal authority to perform the activities or procedures discussed. Such specific determination should be made only with the aid of legal counsel. Some images in this book feature models. These models do not necessarily endorse, represent, or participate in the activities represented in the images. THE PUBLISHER MAKES NO REPRESENTATIONS OR WARRANTIES OF ANY KIND, WHETHER EXPRESS OR IMPLIED, WITH RESPECT TO THE CONTENT HEREIN. THIS PUBLICATION IS PROVIDED AS-IS, AND THE PUBLISHER AND ITS AFFILIATES SHALL NOT BE LIABLE FOR ANY ACTUAL, INCIDENTAL, SPECIAL, CONSEQUENTIAL, PUNITIVE, OR EXEMPLARY DAMAGES RESULTING, IN WHOLE OR IN PART, FROM THE READER'S USE OF, OR RELIANCE UPON, SUCH CONTENT.

User's Guide

Welcome to the Assessment Technologies Institute® Nursing Leadership and Management Review Module Edition 6.0. The mission of ATI's Content Mastery Series® review modules is to provide user-friendly compendiums of nursing knowledge that will:

- Help you locate important information quickly.

- Assist in your learning efforts.

- Provide exercises for applying your nursing knowledge.

- Facilitate your entry into the nursing profession as a newly licensed nurse.

Organization

Chapters in this review module use a nursing concepts organizing framework, beginning with an overview describing the central concept and its relevance to nursing. Subordinate themes are covered in outline form to demonstrate relationships and present the information in a clear, succinct manner. Each chapter is divided into sections that group related concepts and contain their own overviews. These sections are included in the table of contents.

Application Exercises

Questions are provided at the end of each chapter so you can practice applying your knowledge. The Application Exercises include NCLEX-style questions, such as multiple-choice and multiple-select items, and questions that ask you to apply your knowledge in other formats, such as by completing an ATI Active Learning Template. After the Application Exercises, an answer key is provided, along with rationales for the answers.

NCLEX® Connections

To prepare for the NCLEX, it is important for you to understand how the content in this review module is connected to the NCLEX test plan. You can find information on the detailed test plan at the National Council of State Boards of Nursing's Web site: https://www.ncsbn.org/. When reviewing content in this review module, regularly ask yourself, "How does this content fit into the test plan, and what types of questions related to this content should I expect?"

To help you in this process, we've included NCLEX Connections at the beginning of each unit and with each question in the Application Exercises Answer Keys. The NCLEX Connections at the beginning of each unit will point out areas of the detailed test plan that relate to the content within that unit. The NCLEX Connections attached to the Application Exercises Answer Keys will demonstrate how each exercise fits within the detailed content outline.

These NCLEX Connections will help you understand how the detailed content outline is organized, starting with major client needs categories and subcategories and followed by related content areas and tasks. The major client needs categories are:

- Safe and Effective Care Environment
  - Management of Care
  - Safety and Infection Control
- Health Promotion and Maintenance
- Psychosocial Integrity
- Physiological Integrity
  - Basic Care and Comfort
  - Pharmacological and Parenteral Therapies
  - Reduction of Risk Potential
  - Physiological Adaptation

An NCLEX Connection might, for example, alert you that content within a unit is related to:

- Management of Care
  - Advance Directives
    - Provide client with information about advance directives.

QSEN Competencies

As you use the review modules, you will note the integration of the Quality and Safety Education for Nurses (QSEN) competencies throughout the chapters. These competencies are integral components of the curriculum of many nursing programs in the United States and prepare you to provide safe, high-quality care as a newly licensed RN. Icons appear to draw your attention to the six QSEN competencies which include:

- Safety: The minimization of risk factors that could cause injury or harm while promoting quality care and maintaining a secure environment for clients, self, and others.
- Patient-Centered Care: The provision of caring and compassionate, culturally sensitive care that addresses clients' physiological, psychological, sociological, spiritual, and cultural needs, preferences, and values.
- Evidence Based Practice: The use of current knowledge from research and other credible sources, on which to base clinical judgment and client care.
- Informatics: The use of information technology as a communication and information-gathering tool that supports clinical decision making and scientifically based nursing practice.
- Quality Improvement: Care related and organizational processes that involve the development and implementation of a plan to improve health care services and better meet clients' needs.
- Teamwork and Collaboration: The delivery of client care in partnership with multidisciplinary members of the health care team, to achieve continuity of care and positive client outcomes.

Icons

Icons are used throughout the review module to draw your attention to particular areas. Keep an eye out for these icons:

 This icon is used for NCLEX connections.

 This icon is used for content related to safety and is a QSEN competency. When you see this icon, take note of safety concerns or steps that nurses can take to ensure client safety and a safe environment.

 This icon is a QSEN competency which indicates the important of a holistic approach to providing care.

 This icon, a QSEN competency, points out the integration of research into clinical practice.

 This icon is a QSEN competency and highlights the use of information technology to support nursing practice.

 This icon is used to focus on the QSEN competency of integrating planning processes to meet clients' needs.

 This icon highlights the QSEN competency of care delivery using an interprofessional approach.

 This icon indicates that a media supplement, such as a graphic, an animation, or a video, is available. If you have an electronic copy of the review module, this icon will appear alongside clickable links to media supplements. If you have a hardcopy version of the review module, visit www.atitesting.com for details on how to access these features.

Feedback

ATI welcomes feedback regarding this review module. Please provide comments to: comments@atitesting.com.

Table of Contents

CHAPTER 1   Managing Client Care

TOPICS

› Leadership and Management
› Critical Thinking
› Assigning, Delegating, and Supervising
› Staff Education
› Quality Improvement
› Performance Appraisal, Peer Review, and Disciplinary Action
› Conflict Resolution
› Resource Management

NCLEX® CONNECTIONS

When reviewing the chapters in this unit, keep in mind the relevant sections of the NCLEX® outline, in particular:

Client Needs: Management of Care

› Relevant topics/tasks include:
  » Case Management
    › Plan safe, cost effective care for the client.
  » Concepts of Management
    › Manage conflict among clients and health care staff.
  » Delegation
    › Evaluate delegated tasks to ensure correct completion of activities.
  » Establishing Priorities
    › Apply knowledge of pathophysiology when establishing priorities for interventions with multiple clients.
  » Performance Improvement
    › Participate in performance improvement/quality assurance processes.
  » Supervision
    › Evaluate the effectiveness of staff member's time management skills.

chapter 1

Overview

- Managing client care requires leadership and management skills and knowledge to effectively coordinate and carry out client care.

- To effectively manage client care, a nurse must develop knowledge and skills in several areas, including:
  - Leadership and Management
  - Critical Thinking, Clinical Reasoning, Clinical Judgment
  - Prioritization and Time Management
  - Assigning, Delegating, and Supervising
  - Staff Education
  - Quality Improvement
  - Performance Appraisal, Peer Review, and Disciplinary Action
  - Conflict Resolution
  - Resource Management

LEADERSHIP AND MANAGEMENT

Overview

- Leadership and management are concepts that are integral to effective management and motivation of staff and clients. In their simplest terms:
  - Management is the process of planning, organizing, directing, and coordinating the work within an organization.
  - Leadership is the ability to inspire others to achieve a desired outcome.

- Effective managers usually possess good leadership skills; however, effective leaders are not always in a management position.

- Managers have formal positions of power and authority; leaders may have only the informal power afforded them by their peers.

- One cannot be a leader without followers.

- A number of theories describe the characteristics of a leader. Behavioral theories describe leadership styles. Transactional and transformational leadership theories contrast two types of leaders. The emotionally intelligent leader displays sensitivity when interacting with others.

Leadership

- Leadership Styles
  - Most can be categorized as authoritative, democratic, or laissez-faire.
    - Authoritative
      - Makes decisions for the group.
      - Motivates by coercion.
      - Communication occurs down the chain of command.
      - Work output by staff is usually high – good for crisis situations and bureaucratic settings.
      - Effective for employees with little or no formal education.
    - Democratic
      - Includes the group when decisions are made.
      - Motivates by supporting staff achievements.
      - Communication occurs up and down the chain of command.
      - Work output by staff is usually of good quality – good when cooperation and collaboration are necessary.
    - Laissez-faire
      - Makes very few decisions, and does little planning.
      - Motivation is largely the responsibility of individual staff members.
      - Communication occurs up and down the chain of command and between group members.
      - Work output is low unless an informal leader evolves from the group.
      - Effective with professional employees.
  - The use of any of these styles may be appropriate depending on the situation.
- Characteristics of Leaders
  - Initiative
  - Inspiration
  - Energy
  - Positive attitude
  - Communication skills
  - Respect
  - Problem-solving and critical-thinking skills
- Leaders have a combination of personality traits and leadership skills.
  - Great leaders were once thought to be born with skills that could not be acquired.
  - Contemporary leadership theory supports the belief that leaders can develop the necessary skills.

- Leaders influence willing followers to move toward a goal.
  - Leaders have goals that may or may not reflect those of the organization.
- Transformational leaders empower followers to assume responsibility for a communal vision, and personal development is a secondary outcome.
- Transactional leaders focus on immediate problems, maintaining the status quo and using rewards to motivate followers.
- Emotional Intelligence
  - Emotional intelligence is the ability of an individual to perceive and manage the emotions of self and others.
  - The nurse must be able to perceive and understand his own emotions and the emotions of the client and family in order to provide client-centered care.
  - Emotional intelligence is also an important characteristic of the successful nurse leader.

  - The emotionally intelligent leader
    - Has insight into the emotions of members of the team.
    - Understands the perspective of others.
    - Encourages constructive criticism and is open to new ideas.
    - Is able to maintain focus while multitasking.
    - Manages emotions and channels them in a positive direction, which in turn helps the team accomplish its goals.
    - Is committed to the delivery of high-quality client care.
    - Refrains from judgment in controversial or emotionally charged situations until facts are gathered.
  - Emotional intelligence is developed through understanding the concept and applying it to practice in everyday situations.

Management

- Characteristics of Managers
  - Hold formal position of authority and power
  - Possess clinical expertise
  - Network with members of the team
  - Coach subordinates
  - Make decisions about organization function, including resources, budget, hiring, and firing
- The five major management functions are planning, organizing, staffing, directing, and controlling.
  - Planning – The decisions regarding what needs to be done, how it will be done, and who is going to do it
  - Organizing – The organizational structure that determines the lines of authority, channels of communication, and where decisions are made

- ○ Staffing – The acquisition and management of adequate staff and staffing mix
- ○ Directing – The leadership role assumed by a manager that influences and motivates staff to perform assigned roles
- ○ Controlling – The evaluation of staff performance and evaluation of unit goals to ensure identified outcomes are being met

CRITICAL THINKING

Overview

- Critical Thinking
  - ○ Critical thinking is used when analyzing client issues and problems. Thinking skills include interpretation, analysis, evaluation, inference and explanation. These skills assist the nurse to determine the most appropriate action to take.
  - ○ Critical thinking reflects upon the meaning of statements, examines available data, and uses reason to make informed decisions.
  - ○ Critical thinking is necessary to reflect and evaluate from a broader scope of view.
  - ○ Sometimes one must think "outside the box" to find solutions that are best for clients, staff, and the organization.
- Clinical Reasoning
  - ○ Clinical reasoning is the mental process used when analyzing the elements of a clinical situation and using analysis to make a decision.
  - ○ Clinical reasoning supports the clinical decision making process by:
    - Guiding the nurse through the process of assessing and compiling data.
    - Selecting and discarding data based on relevance.
    - Using nursing knowledge to make decisions about client care. Problem solving is a part of decision making.
- Clinical Judgment
  - ○ Clinical judgment is the decision made regarding a course of action based on a critical analysis of data when using knowledge is applied to a clinical situation.
    - The nurse uses clinical judgment to:
      - □ Analyze data and related evidence.
      - □ Ascertain the meaning of the data and evidence.
      - □ Determine client outcomes desired and/or achieved as indicated by evidence-based practices.

Prioritization and Time Management

- Nurses must continuously set and reset priorities in order to meet the needs of multiple clients and to maintain client safety.
- Priority setting requires that decisions be made regarding the order in which:
  - Clients are seen.
  - Assessments are completed.
  - Interventions are provided.
  - Steps in a client procedure are completed.
  - Components of client care are completed.
- Establishing priorities in nursing practice requires that these decisions be made based on evidence obtained:
  - During shift reports and other communications with members of the health care team.
  - Through careful review of documents.
  - By continuously and accurately collecting client data.

PRIORITIZATION PRINCIPLES IN CLIENT CARE	
Principle	Examples
› Prioritize systemic before local ("life before limb").	› Prioritizing interventions for a client in shock over interventions for a client with a localized limb injury
› Prioritize acute (less opportunity for physical adaptation) before chronic (greater opportunity for physical adaptation).	› Prioritizing the care of a client with a new injury/illness (e.g., mental confusion, chest pain) or an acute exacerbation of a previous illness over the care of a client with a long-term chronic illness
› Prioritize actual problems before potential future problems.	› Prioritizing administration of medication to a client experiencing acute pain over ambulation of a client at risk for thrombophlebitis
› Listen carefully to clients and don't assume.	› Recognizing that a postoperative client's report of pain could be due to pain in another location rather than expected surgical pain
› Recognize and respond to trends versus transient findings.	› Recognizing a gradual deterioration in a client's level of consciousness and/or Glasgow Coma Scale score
› Recognize signs of medical emergencies and complications versus "expected client findings."	› Recognizing signs of increasing intracranial pressure in a client newly diagnosed with a stroke versus the clinical findings expected following a stroke
› Apply clinical knowledge to procedural standards to determine the priority action.	› Recognizing that the timing of administration of antidiabetic and antimicrobial medications is more important than administration of some other medications

- Priority Setting Frameworks
  - Maslow's Hierarchy
    - The nurse should consider this hierarchy of human needs when prioritizing interventions. For example, the nurse should prioritize a client's:
      - Need for airway, oxygenation (or breathing), circulation, and potential for disability over need for shelter.
      - Need for a safe and secure environment over a need for family support.

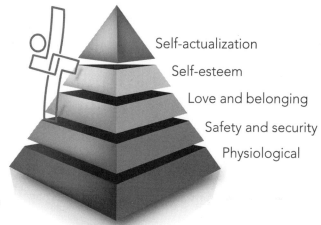

Self-actualization

Self-esteem

Love and belonging

Safety and security

Physiological

  - Airway Breathing Circulation (ABC) Framework
    - The ABC framework identifies, in order, the three basic needs for sustaining life:
      - An open airway is necessary for breathing, so it is the highest priority.
      - Breathing is necessary for oxygenation of the blood to occur.
      - Circulation is necessary for oxygenated blood to reach the body's tissues.
    - The severity of clinical manifestations should also be considered when determining priorities. A severe circulation problem may take priority over a minor breathing problem.
    - Some frameworks also include a "D" for disability, addressing the high priority given for prevention of disabilities.

PRIORITY	ASSESSMENT	INTERVENTIONS
First	› Airway	› Identify an airway concern (obstruction, stridor). › Establish a patent airway if indicated. › Recognize that 3 to 5 min without oxygen causes irreversible brain damage secondary to cerebral anoxia.
Second	› Breathing	› Assess the effectiveness of the client's breathing (apnea, depressed respiratory rate). › Intervene as appropriate (reposition, administer naloxone [Narcan]).
Third	› Circulation	› Identify circulation concern (hypotension, dysrhythmia, inadequate cardiac output, compartment syndrome). › Institute appropriate actions to reverse or minimize circulatory alteration.
Fourth	› Disability	› Assess for current or evolving disability (neurological deficits, stroke in evolution). › Implement action to slow down development of disability.

- ○ Safety/Risk Reduction
  - ▪ Look first for a safety risk. For example, is there a finding that suggests a risk for airway obstruction, hypoxia, bleeding, infection, or injury?
  - ▪ Next ask, "What's the risk to the client?" and "How significant is the risk compared to other posed risks?"
  - ▪ Give priority to responding to whatever finding poses the greatest (or most imminent) risk to the client's physical well-being.
- ○ Assessment/Data Collection First
  - ▪ Use the nursing process to gather pertinent information prior to making a decision regarding a plan of action. For example, determine if additional information is needed prior to calling the provider to ask for pain medication for a client.
- ○ Survival Potential
  - ▪ Use this framework for situations in which health resources are extremely limited (mass casualty, disaster triage).
  - ▪ Give priority to clients who have a reasonable chance of survival with prompt intervention. Clients who have a limited likelihood of survival even with intense intervention are assigned the lowest priority.
- ○ Least Restrictive/Least Invasive
  - ▪ Select interventions that maintain client safety while posing the least amount of restriction to the client. For example, if a client with a high fall risk index is getting out of bed without assistance, move the client closer to the nurses' work area rather than choosing to apply restraints.
  - ▪ Select interventions that are the least invasive. For example, bladder training for the incontinent client is a better option than an indwelling urinary catheter.
- ○ Acute vs. Chronic/Urgent vs. Nonurgent/Stable vs. Unstable
  - ▪ A client who has an acute problem takes priority over a client who has a chronic problem.
  - ▪ A client who has an urgent need takes priority over a client who has a nonurgent need.
  - ▪ A client who has unstable findings takes priority over a client who has stable findings.

Time Management

- • Good time management
  - ○ Facilitates greater productivity.
  - ○ Decreases work-related stress.
  - ○ Helps ensure the provision of quality and appropriately prioritized client care.
  - ○ Enhances satisfaction with care provided.
- • Poor time management
  - ○ Impairs productivity.
  - ○ Leads to feelings of being overwhelmed and stressed.
  - ○ Increases omission of important tasks.
  - ○ Creates dissatisfaction with care provided.

- Time management involves organizing care according to client care needs and priorities.
  - What must be done immediately (administration of analgesic or antiemetic, assessment of unstable client)?
  - What must be done by a specific time to ensure client safety, quality care, and compliance with facility policies and procedures (medication administration, vital signs, blood glucose monitoring)?
  - What must be done by the end of the shift (ambulation of the client, discharge and/or discharge teaching, dressing change)?
  - What can be delegated?
    - What can be done only by an RN?
    - What client care responsibilities can be delegated to other health care team members, such as licensed practical nurses (LPNs) and assistive personnel (AP)?
    - How can scheduled client care activities most efficiently be shared by these two groups of care providers?
- Time management involves using time-saving strategies and avoiding time wasters.

TIME SAVERS	TIME WASTERS
› Documenting nursing interventions as soon as possible after completion to facilitate accurate and thorough documentation	› Documenting at the end of the shift all client care provided and assessments done
› Grouping activities that are to be performed on the same client or are in close physical proximity to prevent unnecessary walking	› Making repeated trips to the supply room for equipment
› Estimating how long each activity will take and planning accordingly	› Providing care as opportunity arises regardless of other responsibilities
› Mentally envisioning the procedure to be performed and ensuring that all equipment has been gathered prior to entering the client's room	› Missing equipment when preparing to perform a procedure
› Taking time to plan care and taking priorities into consideration	› Failing to plan or managing by crisis
› Delegating activities to other staff when client care workload is beyond what can be handled by one nurse	› Being reluctant to delegate or underdelegating
› Enlisting the aid of other staff when a team approach would be more efficient than an individual approach	› Not asking for help when needed or trying to provide all client care independently
› Completing more difficult or strenuous tasks when energy level is high	› Procrastinating – delaying time-consuming, less desirable tasks until late in the shift
› Avoiding interruptions and graciously but assertively saying "no" to unreasonable or poorly timed requests for help	› Agreeing to help other team members when time is already compromised
› Setting a realistic standard for completion of care and level of performance within the constraints of assignment and resources	› Setting unrealistic standards for completion of care and level of performance within constraints of assignment and resources

TIME SAVERS	TIME WASTERS
› Completing one task before beginning another task	› Starting several tasks at once and not completing tasks before starting others
› Breaking large tasks into smaller tasks to make them more manageable	› Not addressing low level of skill competency, increasing time on task
› Using an organizational sheet to plan care	› Providing care without a written plan
› Using breaks to socialize with staff	› Socializing with staff during client care time

- Time management is a cyclic process.
  - ○ Time initially spent developing a plan will save time later and help to avoid management by crisis.
  - ○ Set goals and plan care based on established priorities and thoughtful utilization of resources.
  - ○ Complete one client care task before beginning the next, starting with the highest priority task.
  - ○ Reprioritize remaining tasks based on continual reassessment of client care needs.
  - ○ At the end of the day, perform a time analysis and determine if time was used wisely.
- Time Management and Teamwork
  - ○ Be cognizant of assistance needed by other health care team members.
  - ○ Offer to help when unexpected crises occur.
  - ○ Assist other team members with provision of care when experiencing a period of "down time."
- Time Management and Self-Care
  - ○ Take time for oneself.
  - ○ Schedule time for breaks and meals.
  - ○ Take physical and mental breaks from work/unit.

ASSIGNING, DELEGATING, AND SUPERVISING

Overview

- Assigning is the process of transferring the authority, accountability, and responsibility of client care to another member of the health care team.
- Delegating is the process of transferring the authority and responsibility to another team member to complete a task, while retaining the accountability.
- Supervising is the process of directing, monitoring, and evaluating the performance of tasks by another member of the health care team. RNs are responsible for the supervision of client care tasks delegated to assistive personnel (AP) and licensed practical nurses (LPNs) – also known, respectively, as unlicensed assistive personnel (UAP) and licensed vocational nurses (LVNs).
  - ○ Licensed personnel are nurses who have completed a course of study, successfully passed either the NCLEX-PN® or NCLEX-RN® exam, and been issued a license by a board of nursing.

- Assistive personnel (AP) are specially trained to function in an assistive role to licensed nurses in client care activities.

    - These individuals may be nursing personnel, such as certified nursing assistants (CNAs) or certified medical assistants (CMAs), or they may be nonnursing personnel to whom nursing activities may be delegated, such as dialysis technicians, monitor technicians, and phlebotomists.

    - Some health care entities may differentiate between nurse and nonnurse assistive personnel by using the acronym NAP for nursing assistive personnel.

- Nurses must delegate appropriately and supervise adequately to ensure that clients receive safe, quality care.
- Delegation decisions are based on individual client needs, facility policies and job descriptions, the state nurse practice act, and professional standards.
- Legal/ethical concerns must be considered when assigning and delegating.
    - The nurse leader should recognize limitations and use available information and resources to make the best possible decisions at the time. The nurse must remember that it is his responsibility to ensure that clients receive safe, effective nursing care.
    - Nurses must follow the ANA codes of standards in delegating and assigning tasks.

Assigning

- Assigning is performed in a downward or lateral manner with regard to members of the health care team.
- Assignment Factors
    - Client factors
        - Condition of the client and level of care needed
        - Specific care needs (cardiac monitoring, mechanical ventilation)
        - Need for special precautions (isolation precautions, fall precautions, seizure precautions)
        - Procedures requiring a significant time commitment
    - Health care team factors
        - Knowledge and skill level of team members
        - Amount of supervision necessary
        - Staffing mix (RNs, LPNs, AP)
        - Nurse-to-client ratio
        - Experience with similar clients
        - Familiarity of staff member with unit
- When a nurse receives an inappropriate assignment, she should take the following actions:
    - Bring the inappropriate assignment to the attention of the scheduling/charge nurse and negotiate a new assignment.
    - If no resolution is arrived at, take the concern up the chain of command.
    - If a satisfactory resolution is still not arrived at, an unsafe staffing complaint in the form of an Assignment Despite Objection (ADO) or Document of Practice Situation (DOPS) should be filed with the appropriate administrator.
    - Failure to accept the assignment without following the proper channels may be considered abandonment.

Delegating and Supervising

- A licensed nurse is responsible for providing clear directions when a task is initially delegated and for periodic reassessment and evaluation of the outcome of the task.
  - RNs may delegate to other RNs, LPNs, and AP.
    - RNs must be knowledgeable about the applicable state nurse practice act and regulations regarding the use of LPNs and AP.
    - RNs must delegate tasks so that they can complete higher level tasks that only RNs can perform. This allows more efficient use of all members of the health care team.
  - LPNs may delegate to other LPNs and AP.
- Delegation Factors
  - Nurses can only delegate tasks appropriate for the skill and education level of the health care provider who is receiving the assignment.
  - RNs cannot delegate the nursing process, client education, or tasks that require clinical judgment to LPNs or AP.
  - Task factors – Prior to delegating client care, the nurse should consider:
    - Predictability of outcome
      - □ Will the completion of the task have a predictable outcome?
      - □ Is it a routine treatment?
      - □ Is it a new treatment?
    - Potential for harm
      - □ Is there a chance that something negative may happen to the client (risk for bleeding, risk for aspiration)?
      - □ Is the client unstable?
    - Complexity of care
      - □ Are complex tasks required as a part of the client's care?
      - □ Is the delegatee legally able to perform the task and does he have the skills necessary?
    - Need for problem solving and innovation
      - □ Will a judgment need to be made while performing the task?
      - □ Does it require nursing assessment skills?
    - Level of interaction with the client
      - □ Is there a need to provide psychosocial support or education during the performance of the task?
  - Delegatee factors – Considerations for selection of an appropriate delegatee include:
    - Education, training, and experience
    - Knowledge and skill to perform the task
    - Level of critical thinking required to complete the task
    - Ability to communicate with others as it pertains to the task

- Demonstrated competence
- The delegatee's culture
- Agency policies and procedures and licensing legislation (state nurse practice acts)

EXAMPLES OF TASKS THAT CAN BE DELEGATED TO LPNS AND AP (PROVIDED AGENCY POLICY AND STATE PRACTICE GUIDELINES PERMIT)	
To LPNs	**To AP**
› Monitoring client findings (as input to the RN's ongoing assessment of the client) › Reinforcement of client teaching from a standard care plan › Tracheostomy care › Suctioning › Checking nasogastric tube patency › Administration of enteral feedings › Insertion of a urinary catheter › Medication administration (excluding intravenous medications in several states)	› Activities of daily living (ADLs) » Bathing » Grooming » Dressing » Toileting » Ambulating » Feeding (without swallowing precautions) » Positioning » Bed making › Specimen collection › Intake and output (I&O) › Vital signs (on stable clients)

- Delegation and Supervision Guidelines
  - Use nursing judgment and knowledge related to the scope of practice and delegatee's skill level when delegating.
  - Use the five rights of delegation
    - What tasks should be delegated (right task)
    - Under what circumstances (right circumstance)
    - To whom (right person)
    - What information should be communicated (right direction/communication)
    - How to supervise/evaluate (right supervision/evaluation)
  - Right task
    - Identify what tasks are appropriate to delegate for each specific client.
      - A right task is repetitive, requires little supervision, and is relatively noninvasive for the client.
    - Delegate tasks to appropriate levels of team members (LPN, AP) based on standards of practice, legal and facility guidelines, and available resources.

RIGHT TASK	WRONG TASK
› Delegate AP to assist a client who has pneumonia to use a bedpan.	› Delegate AP to administer a nebulizer treatment to a client who has pneumonia.

- ○ Right circumstance
  - Assess the health status and complexity of care required by the client.
  - Match the complexity of care demands to the skill level of the health care team member.
  - Consider the workload of the team member.

RIGHT CIRCUMSTANCE	WRONG CIRCUMSTANCE
› Delegate AP to assist in obtaining vital signs from a stable postoperative client.	› Delegate AP to assist in obtaining vital signs from a postoperative client who required naloxone (Narcan) for depressed respirations.

- ○ Right person
  - Assess and verify the competency of the health care team member.
    - □ The task must be within the team member's scope of practice.
    - □ The team member must have the necessary competence/training.
  - Continually review the performance of the team member and determine care competency.
  - Assess team member performance based on standards and, when necessary, take steps to remediate a failure to meet standards.

RIGHT PERSON	WRONG PERSON
› Delegate LPN to administer enteral feedings to a client who has a head injury.	› Delegate AP to administer enteral feedings to a client who has a head injury.

- ○ Right direction/communication
  - Communicate either in writing or orally:
    - □ Data that need to be collected
    - □ Method and time line for reporting, including when to report concerns/assessment findings
    - □ Specific task(s) to be performed; client-specific instructions
    - □ Expected results, time lines, and expectations for follow-up communication

RIGHT DIRECTION/COMMUNICATION	WRONG DIRECTION/COMMUNICATION
› Delegate AP the task of assisting the client in room 312 with a shower, to be completed by 0900.	› Delegate AP the task of assisting the client in room 312 with morning hygiene.

- ○ Right supervision/evaluation
  - The delegating nurse must:
    - □ Provide supervision, either directly or indirectly (assigning supervision to another licensed nurse).
    - □ Provide clear directions and understandable expectations of the task(s) to be performed (time frames, what to report).
    - □ Monitor performance.
    - □ Provide feedback.

- ▢ Intervene if necessary (unsafe clinical practice).

- ▢ Evaluate the client and determine if client outcomes were met.

- ▢ Evaluate client care tasks and identify needs for quality improvement activities and/or additional resources.

RIGHT SUPERVISION	WRONG SUPERVISION
› After completing the admission assessment, an RN delegates to an AP the task of ambulating a client.	› Prior to performing an admission assessment, an RN delegates to an AP the task of ambulating a client.

- Supervision occurs after delegation. A supervisor oversees a staff's performance of delegated activities and determines if:

  - ○ Completion of tasks is on schedule.

  - ○ Performance was at a satisfactory level.

  - ○ Abnormal or unexpected findings were documented and reported.

  - ○ Assistance is needed to complete assigned tasks in a timely manner.

  - ○ Assignment should be re-evaluated and possibly changed.

STAFF EDUCATION

Overview

- Staff education refers to the nurse's involvement in the orientation, socialization, education, and training of fellow health care workers to ensure the competence of all staff and to help them meet standards set forth by the facility and accrediting bodies. The process of staff education may also be referred to as staff development.

- The quality of client care provided is directly related to the education and level of competency of health care providers.

- The nurse leader has a responsibility in maintaining competent staff.

- Nurse leaders work with a unique, diverse workforce. Diversity should be respected and recognized.

Orientation

- Orientation helps newly licensed nurses translate the knowledge, skills, and attitudes learned in nursing school into practice.

- Orientation to the Institution

  - ○ The newly licensed nurse is introduced to the philosophy, mission, and goals of the institution and department.

  - ○ Policies and procedures that are based on institutional standards are reviewed.

  - ○ Use of and access to the institution's computer system is a significant focus.

  - ○ Safety and security protocols are emphasized in relation to the nurse's role.

- Orientation to the Unit
  - ○ Classroom orientation usually moves onto the unit and is continued with an assigned preceptor.
  - ○ Preceptors assist in orienting newly licensed nurses to a unit and supervising their performance and acquisition of skills.
  - ○ Preceptors are usually assigned to newly licensed nurses for a limited amount of time.
  - ○ Mentors may also serve as a newly licensed nurse's preceptor, but their relationship usually lasts longer and focuses more on assumption of the professional role and relationships, as well as socialization to practice.
  - ○ Coaches establish a collaborative relationship to help a nurse establish individual goals. The relationship is typically time limited.

Socialization

- Socialization is the process by which a person learns a new role and the values and culture of the group within which that role will be implemented.
  - ○ Successful socialization helps new staff members fit in with already established staff on a client care unit.
  - ○ Staff development educators and unit managers may begin this process during interviewing and orientation.
  - ○ Nurse preceptors/mentors are frequently used to assist newly licensed nurses with this process on the clinical unit.

Education and Training

- Staff education, or staff development, is the process by which a staff member gains knowledge and skills. The goal of staff education is to ensure that staff members have and maintain the most current knowledge and skills necessary to meet the needs of clients.

STAFF EDUCATION CHARACTERISTICS	IDENTIFIED AND/OR PROVIDED BY
› Involves methods appropriate to learning domain and learning styles of staff.	› Peers, unit managers, staff development educators
› Initiated in specific situations » New policies or procedures implemented » New equipment becomes available » Educational need identified	› Unit managers, staff development educators
› May focus on one-on-one approach	› Unit manager, charge nurse, preceptor
› Can use "just in time" training to meet immediate needs for client care	› Staff members, supervisors
› Higher education degree or certification	› Staff

- Educational programs should be provided using the sequence below:

STEPS IN PROVIDING EDUCATIONAL PROGRAMS	
1. Identify and respond	› To identify need for knowledge or skill proficiency
2. Analyze	› Deficiencies, and develop learning objectives to meet need
3. Research	› Resources available to address learning objectives
4. Plan	› Program to address objectives using available resources
5. Implement	› Program(s) at time conducive to staff attendance; consider online learning modules
6. Evaluate	› Use materials and observations to measure behavior changes secondary to learning objectives

- An increase in knowledge and competence is the goal of staff education.
  - Competence is the ability of an employee to meet the requirements of a particular role at an established level of performance. Nurses will usually progress through several stages of proficiency as they gain experience in a particular area.
  - Patricia Benner (1984) identified five stages of nursing ability, which are based on level of competence. Level of competence is directly related to length of time in practice and exposure to clinical situations. When nurses move to a new clinical setting that requires acquisition of new skills and knowledge, their level of competence will return to a lower stage.

FIVE STAGES OF NURSING ABILITY	
Novice nurse	› Novice nurses may be students or newly licensed nurses with minimal clinical experience. Approach situations from theoretical perspective relying on context-free facts and established guidelines. Rules govern practice.
Advanced beginner	› Most new nurses function at the level of the advanced beginner. Practice independently in the performance of many tasks and can make some clinical judgments. Begin to rely on prior experience to make practice decisions.
Competent nurse	› These are usually nurses who have been in practice for 2 to 3 years. Demonstrate increasing levels of skill and proficiency and clinical judgment. Exhibit the ability to organize and plan care using abstract and analytical thinking. Can anticipate the long-term outcomes of personal actions.
Proficient nurse	› These are nurses who have a significant amount of experience upon which to base their practice. Enhanced observational abilities allow nurses to be able to conceptualize situations more holistically. Well-developed critical thinking and decision-making skills allow nurses to recognize and respond to unexpected changes.
Expert nurse	› Expert nurses have garnered a wealth of experience so they can view situations holistically and process information efficiently. Make decisions using an advanced level of intuition and analytical ability. Do not need to rely on rules to comprehend a situation and take action.

http://www.scribd.com/doc/27103958/Benner-Theory-Novice-to-Expert

QUALITY IMPROVEMENT

Overview

- Quality improvement (performance improvement, quality control) is the process used to identify and resolve performance deficiencies. Quality improvement includes measuring performance against a set of predetermined standards. In health care these standards may be set by the specific facility and take into consideration accrediting and professional standards.

- Standards of care that are established should reflect optimal goals and be based on evidence.

- The quality improvement process focuses on assessment of outcomes and determines ways to improve the delivery of quality care. All levels of employees are involved in the quality improvement process.

- The Joint Commission's accreditation standards require institutions to show evidence of quality improvement in order to attain accreditation status.

Quality Improvement Process

- The quality improvement process begins with identification of standards and outcome indicators based on evidence.

  - Outcome, or clinical, indicators reflect desired client outcomes related to the standard under review.

  - Structure indicators reflect the setting in which care is being provided and the available human and material resources.

  - Process indicators reflect how client care is provided and are established by policies and procedures (clinical practice guidelines).

  - Benchmarks are goals that are set to determine at what level the outcome indicators should be met.

    - While process indicators provide important information about how a procedure is being carried out, an outcome indicator measures whether that procedure is effective in meeting the desired benchmark. For example: the use of incentive spirometers in postoperative clients may be determined to be 92% (process indicator) but the rate of postoperative pneumonia may be determined to be 8% (outcome indicator). If the benchmark is set at 5%, the benchmark for that outcome indicator is not being met and the structure and process variables need to be analyzed to identify potential areas for improvement.

- Steps in the Quality Improvement Process

  - A standard is developed and approved by facility committee.

  - Standards are made available to employees by way of policies and procedures.

  - Quality issues are identified by staff, management, or risk management department.

  - An interprofessional team is developed to review the issue.

  - The current state of structure and process related to the issue is analyzed.

- Data collection methods are determined.
  - Quantitative methods are primarily used in the data collection process, although client interview is also an option.
  - Audits can produce valuable quantitative data. There are several types of audits.
    - Types of Audits
      - Structure audits evaluate the influence of elements that exist separate from or outside of the client-staff interaction.
      - Process audits review how care was provided and assume a relationship exists between nurses and the quality of care provided.
      - Outcome audits determine what results, if any, occurred as a result of the nursing care provided.
      - Some outcomes are influenced by aspects of care such as the quality of medical care, the level of commitment of managerial staff, and the characteristics of facility's policies and procedures.
      - Nursing-sensitive outcomes are those that are directly affected by the quality of nursing care. Examples include client fall rates and the incidence of nosocomial infections.
    - Timing of Audits
      - Retrospective audits occur after the client receives care.
      - Concurrent audits occur while the client is receiving care.
      - Prospective audits predict how future client care will be affected by current level of services.
- Data is collected, analyzed, and compared with the established benchmark.
- If the benchmark is not met, possible influencing factors are determined. A root cause analysis may be done to critically assess all factors that influence the issue.
  - Root cause analyses focus on variables that surround the consequence of an action or occurrence.
  - Root cause analyses are commonly done for sentinel events (client death, client care resulting in serious physical injury) but may also be done as part of the quality improvement process.

  - A root cause analysis:
    - Investigates the consequence and possible causes.
    - Analyzes the possible causes and relationships that may exist.
    - Determines additional influences at each level of relationship.
    - Determines the root cause or causes.
- Potential solutions or corrective actions are analyzed and one is selected for implementation.
- Educational or corrective action is implemented.
- The issue is reevaluated at a preestablished time to determine the efficacy of the solution or corrective action.

- The Nurse's Role in Quality Improvement
  - ○ Serve as unit representative on committees developing policies and procedures. Use reliable resources for information (Centers for Disease Control and Prevention, professional journals, evidenced-based research).
  - ○ Enhance knowledge and understanding of the facility's policies and procedures.
  - ○ Provide client care consistent with these policies and procedures.
  - ○ Document client care thoroughly and according to facility guidelines.
  - ○ Participate in the collection of information/data related to staff's adherence to selected policy or procedure.
  - ○ Assist with analysis of the information/data.
  - ○ Compare results with the established benchmark.
  - ○ Make a judgment about performance in regard to the findings.
  - ○ Assist with provision of education or training necessary to improve the performance of staff.
  - ○ Act as a role model by practicing in accordance with the established standard.
  - ○ Assist with re-evaluation of staff performance by collection of information/data at a specified time.

PERFORMANCE APPRAISAL, PEER REVIEW, AND DISCIPLINARY ACTION

Overview

- A performance appraisal is the process by which a supervisor evaluates an employee's performance in relation to the job description for that employee's position as well as other expectations the facility may have.
- Performance appraisals are done at regular intervals and may be more frequent for new employees.
- Performance expectations should be based on the standards set forth in a job description and written in objective terms.
- Performance appraisals allow nurses the opportunity to discuss personal goals with the unit manager as well as to receive feedback regarding level of performance. Performance appraisals can also be used as a motivational tool.
- Deficiencies identified during a performance appraisal or reported by coworkers may need to be addressed in a disciplinary manner.

Performance Appraisal and Peer Review

- A formal system for conducting performance appraisals should be in place and used consistently. Performance appraisal tools should reflect the staff member's job description and may be based on various types of scales or surveys.
- Various sources of data should be collected to ensure an unbiased and thorough evaluation of an employee's performance.
  - ○ Data should be collected over time and not just represent isolated incidents.
  - ○ Actual observed behavior should be documented/used as evidence of satisfactory or unsatisfactory performance. These may be called anecdotal notes and are kept in the unit manager or equivalent position's files.

- ○ Peers can be a valuable source of data. Peer review is the evaluation of a colleague's practice by another peer. Peer review should:
  - Begin with an orientation of staff to the peer review process, their professional responsibility in regard to promoting growth of colleagues, and the disposition of data collected.
  - Focus on the peer's performance in relation to the job description or an appraisal tool that is based on institutional standards.
  - Be shared with the peer and usually the manager.
  - Be only part of the data used when completing a staff member's performance appraisal.
  - ○ The employee should be given the opportunity to provide input into the evaluation.
- The performance appraisal review should be hosted by the unit manager in a private setting and held at a time conducive to the staff member's attendance. The unit manager should review the data with the staff member and provide the opportunity for feedback. Personal goals of the staff member should be discussed and documented, and avenues for attainment discussed. Staff members who do not agree with the unit manager's evaluation of their performance should have the opportunity to make written comments on the evaluation form and appeal the rating.

Disciplinary Action

- Deficiencies identified during a performance appraisal or the course of employment should be presented in writing, and corrective action should be based on institutional policy regarding disciplinary actions and/or termination of employment. Evidence regarding the deficiency must support such a claim.
- Some offenses such as mistreatment of a client or use of alcohol or drugs while working warrant immediate dismissal. Lesser infractions should follow a stepwise manner, giving the staff member the opportunity to correct unacceptable behavior.

INFRACTIONS	STEPS IN PROGRESSIVE DISCIPLINE
First	› Informal reprimand › Manager and employee meet » Discuss the issue » Suggestions for improvement/correction
Second	› Written warning › Manager meets with employee to distribute written warning » Review of specific rules/policy violations » Discussion of potential consequences if infractions continue
Third	› Employee placed on suspension with or without pay. Time away from work gives the employee opportunity to: » Examine the issues » Consider alternatives
Fourth	› Employee termination » Follows after multiple warning have been given and employee continues to violate rules and policies

- Staff members who witness an inappropriate action by a coworker should report the infraction up the chain of command. At the time of the infraction, this may be the charge nurse. The unit manager should also be notified, and written documentation by the manager may be placed in the staff member's permanent file.

CONFLICT RESOLUTION

Overview

- Conflict is the result of opposing thoughts, ideas, feelings, perceptions, behaviors, values, opinions, or actions between individuals

- Conflict is an inevitable part of professional, social, and personal life and can have constructive or destructive results. Nurses must understand conflict and how to manage it.

- Problem-solving and negotiation strategies can often be used to prevent a problem from evolving into a conflict.

- Lack of conflict can create organizational stasis, while too much conflict can be demoralizing, produce anxiety, and contribute to burnout.

Categories of Conflict

- Intrapersonal conflict occurs within the person and may involve internal struggle related to contradictory values or wants.
  - Example: A nurse wants to move up on the career ladder but is finding that time with her family is subsequently compromised.

- Interpersonal conflict occurs between two or more people with differing values, goals, and/or beliefs.
  - Interpersonal conflict in the health care setting involves disagreement among nurses, clients, family members, and within a health care team.
  - This is a significant issue in nursing, especially in relation to new nurses, who bring new personalities and perspectives to various health care settings.
  - Interpersonal conflict contributes to burnout and work-related stress.
    - Example: A new nurse is given a client assignment that is heavier than those of other nurses, and when he asks for help, it is denied.
  - Intergroup conflict occurs between two or more groups of individuals, departments, or organizations and may be caused by a new policy or procedure, a change in leadership, or a change in organizational structure.
    - Example: There is confusion as to whether it is the responsibility of the nursing unit or dietary department to pass meal trays.

Organizational Conflict

- Organizational conflict can disrupt working relationships and create a stressful atmosphere.
- If conflict exists to the level that productivity and quality of care are compromised, the unit manager must attempt to identify the origin of the conflict and attempt to resolve it.
- Common causes of organizational conflict include:
  - Ineffective communication
  - Unclear expectations of team members in their various roles
  - Poorly defined or actualized organizational structure
  - Conflicts of interest and variance in standards
  - Incompatibility of individuals
  - Management or staffing changes
  - Diversity related to age, gender, race, or ethnicity

Conflict Resolution Strategies

- Problem Solving
  - Open communication among staff and between staff and clients can help defray the need for conflict resolution.
  - When potential sources of conflict exist, the use of open communication and problem-solving strategies can be effective tools to de-escalate the situation. Actions the nurse can take to promote open communication and de-escalate a conflict include the following:
    - Use "I" statements, and remember to focus on the problem, not on personal differences.
    - Listen carefully to what the other people are saying, and try to understand their perspective.
    - Move a conflict that is escalating to a private location or postpone the discussion until a later time to give everyone a chance to regain control of their emotions.
    - Share ground rules with participants. For example, everyone is to be treated with respect, only one person can speak at a time, and everyone should have a chance to speak.
  - Steps of the problem-solving process
    - Identify the problem – State it in objective terms, minimizing emotional overlay.
    - Discuss possible solutions – Brainstorming solutions as a group may stimulate new solutions to old problems. Encourage individuals to "think outside the box."
    - Analyze identified solutions – The potential pros and cons of each possible solution should be discussed in an attempt to narrow down the number of viable solutions.
    - Select a solution – Based on this analysis, select a solution for implementation.
    - Implement the selected solution – A procedure and time line for implementation should accompany the implementation of the selected solution.
    - Evaluate the solution's ability to resolve the original problem. The outcomes surrounding the new solution should be evaluated according to the predetermined time line. The solution should be given adequate time to become established as a new routine before it is evaluated. If the solution is deemed unsuccessful, the problem-solving process will need to be reinstituted and the problem discussed again.

- Negotiation
  - Negotiation is the process by which interested parties:
    - Resolve ongoing conflicts.
    - Agree on steps to take.
    - Bargain to protect individual or collective interests.
    - Pursue outcomes that benefit mutual interests.
  - Most nurses use negotiation on a daily basis.
  - Negotiation may involve the use of several conflict resolution strategies.
  - The focus is on a win-win solution or a win/lose-win/lose solution in which both parties win and lose a portion of their original objectives.
    - Each party agrees to give up something and the emphasis is on accommodating differences rather than similarities between parties.
    - For example, one nurse offers to care for Client A today if the other will care for Client B tomorrow.

STRATEGY	CHARACTERISTICS
Avoiding/ Withdrawing	› Both parties know there is a conflict, but they refuse to face it or work toward a resolution. › May be appropriate for minor conflicts or when one party holds more power than the other party or if the issue may work itself out over time. › Because the conflict remains, it may surface again at a later date and escalate over time. › This is usually a lose-lose solution.
Smoothing	› One party attempts to "smooth" another party by trying to satisfy the other party. › Often used to preserve or maintain a peaceful work environment. › The focus may be on what is agreed upon, leaving conflict largely unresolved. › This is usually a lose-lose solution.
Competing/ Coercing	› One party pursues a desired solution at the expense of others. › Managers may use this when a quick or unpopular decision must be made. › The party who loses something may experience anger, aggravation, and a desire for retribution. › This is usually a win-lose solution.
Cooperating/ Accommodating	› One party sacrifices something, allowing the other party to get what it wants. This is the opposite of competing. › The original problem may not actually be resolved. › The solution may contribute to future conflict. › This is a lose-win solution.
Compromising/ Negotiating	› Each party gives up something. › To consider this a win/lose-win/lose solution, both parties must give up something equally important. If one party gives up more than the other, it can become a win-lose solution.

○ Consider the following example:

An experienced nurse on a urology unit arrives to work on the night shift. The unit manager immediately asks the nurse to float to a pediatrics unit because the hospital census is high and they are understaffed. The nurse has always maintained a positive attitude when asked to work on another medical-surgical unit but states she does not feel comfortable in the pediatric setting. The manager insists the nurse is the most qualified.

STRATEGY	CHARACTERISTICS
Avoiding/ Withdrawing	› The nurse basically cannot use these strategies due to the immediacy of the situation. The assignment cannot be simply avoided or smoothed over; it must be accepted or rejected.
Competing/ Coercing	› If the nurse truly feels unqualified to work on the pediatric unit, then this approach may be appropriate – the nurse must win and the manager must lose. › Although risking termination by refusing the assignment, the nurse should take an assertive approach and inform the manager that children would be placed at risk.
Cooperating/ Accommodating	› If the nurse decides to accommodate the manager's request, then the children may be at risk for incompetent care. › Practice liability is another issue for consideration.
Compromising/ Negotiating	› This approach generally minimizes the losses for all involved while making certain each party gains something. › For example, the nurse might offer to work on another medical-surgical unit if someone from that unit feels comfortable in the pediatric environment. › Although each party is giving up something (the manager gives in to a different solution and the nurse still has to work on another unit), this sort of compromise can result in a win-win resolution.

Assertive Communication

- Use of assertive communication may be necessary during conflict negotiation.
- Assertive communication allows expression in direct, honest, and nonthreatening ways that do not infringe upon the rights of others.
- It is a communication style that acknowledges and deals with conflict, recognizes others as equals, and provides a direct statement of feelings.
- Elements of assertive communication include:
  ○ Selection of an appropriate location for the verbal exchange
  ○ Maintenance of eye contact
  ○ Establishing trust
  ○ Being sensitive to cultural needs
  ○ Speaking using "I" statements and including affective elements of the situation
  ○ Avoiding using "you" statements that can indicate blame
  ○ Stating concerns using open, honest, and direct statements
  ○ Conveying empathy
  ○ Focusing on the behavior or issue of conflict and avoiding personal attacks
  ○ Concluding with a statement that describes a fair solution

Grievances

- A grievance is a wrong perceived by an employee based on a feeling of unfair treatment that is considered grounds for a formal complaint.
- Grievances that cannot be satisfactorily resolved between the parties involved may need to be managed by a third party.
- All health care facilities have a formal grievance policy that should be followed when a conflict cannot be resolved.
- The steps of an institution's grievance procedure should be outlined in the grievance policy.
- Typical steps of the grievance process include:
  - Formal presentation of the complaint(s) using the proper chain of command
  - Formal hearing if the issue is not resolved at a lower level
  - Professional mediation if a solution is not reached during a formal hearing

RESOURCE MANAGEMENT

Overview

- Resource management includes budgeting and resource allocation. Human, financial, and material resources must be considered.
  - Budgeting is usually the responsibility of the unit manager, but staff nurses may be asked to provide input.
  - Resource allocation is a responsibility of the unit manager as well as every practicing nurse.
  - Providing cost-effective client care should not compromise quality of care.

- Resources (supplies, equipment, personnel) are critical to accomplishing the goals and objectives of a health care facility, so it is essential for nurses to understand how to effectively manage resources.

Cost-Effective Resource Management

- Cost-effective resource allocation includes:
  - Using all levels of personnel to their fullest when making assignments.
  - Providing necessary equipment and properly charging clients.
  - Returning uncontaminated, unused equipment to the appropriate department for credit.
  - Using equipment properly to prevent wastage.
  - Providing training to staff unfamiliar with equipment.
  - Returning equipment (IV, kangaroo pumps) to the proper department (central service, central distribution) as soon as it is no longer needed. This action will prevent further cost to clients.

APPLICATION EXERCISES

1. A nurse receives a change-of-shift report at 0700 for an assigned caseload of clients. Number the following clients in the order in which they should be seen.

_____ A client who has been receiving a blood transfusion since 0400

_____ A client who has an every 4 hr PRN analgesic prescription and who last received pain medication at 0430

_____ A client who is scheduled for a colonoscopy at 1130 and whose informed consent needs to be verified

_____ A client who needs rapid onset insulin before the breakfast trays arrive

_____ A client who is being discharged today and needs reinforcement of teaching regarding dressing changes

2. An older adult client who is on fall precautions is found lying on the floor of his hospital room. Which of the following actions is most appropriate for the nurse to take first?

A. Call the client's provider.

B. Ask a staff member for assistance getting the client back in bed.

C. Inspect the client for injuries.

D. Ask the client why he got out of bed without assistance.

3. A nurse is preparing to initiate IV therapy for a client who has a prescription for morphine 10 mg IV bolus. Using time management principles, which of the following actions should the nurse take first?

A. Mentally envision the procedure when collecting supplies.

B. Enter the room and perform hand hygiene.

C. Eject excessive medication from the prefilled syringe

D. Explain the procedure to the client.

4. An RN on a medical-surgical unit is making assignments at the beginning of the shift. Which of the following tasks should the nurse delegate to the LPN?

A. Obtaining vital signs for a client who is 2 hr postprocedure following a cardiac catheterization

B. Administering a unit of packed red blood cells (RBCs)

C. Instructing a client in the performance of wound care

D. Developing a plan of care for a newly admitted client

5. An LPN ending her shift reports to the RN that a newly hired assistive personnel has not calculated the intake and output for several clients. Which of the following actions should the RN take?

    A. Complete an incident report.

    B. Delegate this task to the LPN.

    C. Ask the AP if assistance is needed to complete the I&O records.

    D. Notify the nurse manager.

6. A nurse manager is developing an orientation plan for newly licensed nurses. Which of the following should the manger include in the plan? (Select all that apply.)

    _____ A. Skill proficiency

    _____ B. Assignment to a preceptor

    _____ C. Budgetary principles

    _____ D. Computerized charting

    _____ E. Socialization into unit culture

    _____ F. Facility policies and procedures

7. A nurse manager is providing information about the audit process to members of the nursing team. Which of the following statements should the nurse manager include? (Select all that apply.)

    _____ A. A structure audit evaluates the setting and resources available to provide care.

    _____ B. An outcome audit evaluates the results of the nursing care provided.

    _____ C. A root cause analysis is indicated when a sentinel event occurs.

    _____ D. Retrospective audits are conducted while the client is receiving care.

    _____ E. After data collection is completed, it is compared to a benchmark.

8. A nurse is participating in a quality improvement study of a procedure frequently performed on the unit. Which of the following will provide the most relevant information regarding the efficacy of the procedure?

    A. Frequency with which procedure is performed

    B. Client satisfaction with performance of procedure

    C. Incidence of complications related to procedure

    D. Accurate documentation of how procedure was performed

9. A nurse is hired to replace a staff member who has resigned. After working on the unit for several weeks, the nurse notices that the unit manager does not intervene when there is conflict between team members, even when it escalates. Which of the following conflict resolution strategies is the unit manager demonstrating?

    A. Avoidance

    B. Smoothing

    C. Cooperating

    D. Negotiating

10. A nurse has received a performance appraisal from the unit manager. Which of the following actions by the unit manager requires intervention?

    A. The evaluation was conducted in the unit manager's office.

    B. Data that was collected for the previous 12 months was presented.

    C. Verbal concerns provided by a staff member were incorporated into the data.

    D. The nurse was asked to review the performance appraisal tool and complete a self-evaluation.

11. A nurse manager is discussing emotional intelligence with the charge nurses on her team. What statements should the manager include in this discussion? Use the Active Learning Template: Basic Concept to complete this item to include the following sections:

    A. Related Content: Definition of emotional intelligence

    B. Underlying Principles: Identify at least three characteristics of an emotionally intelligent leader

APPLICATION EXERCISES KEY

1. **1** The first action the nurse should take is to attend to the client who is receiving blood. It has been 3 hr since the transfusion was initiated, and it should be completed within 4 hr. The client is also at risk for a transfusion reaction; therefore, this is the first action the nurse should take.

    3 Next the nurse should administer PRN pain medication to the client who was last medicated at 0430.

    4 Then the nurse should verify that the informed consent is completed in sufficient time to take any actions needed prior to the scheduled colonoscopy.

    2 The next action the nurse should take is to administer the insulin, which is scheduled to be administered before 0800.

    5 Finally, the nurse should reinforce teaching for the client who is to be discharged and has a prescription for dressing changes.

    Ⓝ NCLEX® Connection: Management of Care, Establishing Priorities

2. A. INCORRECT: The nurse should notify the provider, but this is not the first action the nurse should take.

    B. INCORRECT: The nurse should seek assistance in returning the client to bed, but this is not the first action the nurse should take.

    C. **CORRECT:** Using the nursing process, the first action the nurse should take is to assess the client. Therefore, the first action the nurse should take is to inspect the client for injury.

    D. INCORRECT: It is important to determine why the client got out of bed without assistance in order to prevent future falls, but this is not the first action the nurse should take.

    Ⓝ NCLEX® Connection: Safety and Infection Control, Reporting of Incident/Event/Irregular Occurrence Variance

3. A. **CORRECT:** The first action the nurse should take is to mentally envision the task to ensure that she has all of the needed supplies to avoid wasting time by having to make another trip to obtain supplies.

    B. INCORRECT: The nurse should perform hand hygiene after she enters the client's room. This is not the first action the nurse should take.

    C. INCORRECT: The nurse should eject excessive medication from the prefilled syringe, but this is not the first action the nurse should take.

    D. INCORRECT: The nurse should explain the procedure immediately prior to performing the task. This is not the first action the nurse should take.

    Ⓝ NCLEX® Connection: Management of Care, Assignment, Delegation and Supervision

4. A. **CORRECT:** It is within the scope of practice of the LPN to monitor a client who is 2 hr post procedure for a cardiac catheterization.

    B. INCORRECT: The RN is responsible for administering blood components including packed RBCs.

    C. INCORRECT: The RN is responsible for client education. It is within the scope of practice of the LPN to reinforce client education.

    D. INCORRECT: The RN is responsible for developing a plan of care for a client. It is within the scope of practice for the LPN to suggest additions to the plan of care.

    Ⓝ NCLEX® Connection: Management of Care, Assignment, Delegation and Supervision

5. A. INCORRECT: An incident report is indicated when a critical incident has occurred. It is not appropriate to complete an incident report in this situation.

    B. INCORRECT: The nurse should not redelegate a task that has already been assigned.

    C. **CORRECT:** The nurse should find out what the AP knows about performing the task and provide education for the AP if indicated.

    D. INCORRECT: The RN is capable of handling the situation; therefore, it is not appropriate to notify the nurse manager.

    Ⓝ NCLEX® Connection: Management of Care, Assignment, Delegation and Supervision

6. A. **CORRECT:** The purpose of orientation is to assist the newly licensed nurse to transition from the role of student to the role of employee and licensed nurse. The nurse manager should include evaluation of skill proficiency and provide additional instruction as indicated.

    B. **CORRECT:** The purpose of orientation is to assist the newly licensed nurse to transition from the role of student to the role of employee and licensed nurse. The nurse manager should include assignment of a preceptor to ease the transition of the newly licensed nurse.

    C. INCORRECT: Budgetary principles are an administrative skill that is usually the reasonability of the unit manager.

    D. **CORRECT:** The purpose of orientation is to assist the newly licensed nurse to transition from the role of student to the role of employee and licensed nurse. The nurse manager should include computerized charting, which is an essential skill for the newly licensed nurse.

    E. **CORRECT:** The purpose of orientation is to assist the newly licensed nurse to transition from the role of student to the role of employee and licensed nurse. The nurse manager should include socialization to unit as a way to ease the transition of the newly licensed nurse.

    F. **CORRECT:** The purpose of orientation is to assist the newly licensed nurse to transition from the role of student to the role of employee and licensed nurse. The nurse manager should include information about facility policies and procedures, which is an essential information for the newly licensed nurse.

    Ⓝ NCLEX® Connection: Management of Care, Collaboration with Interdisciplinary Team

7. A. **CORRECT:** A structure audit evaluates the setting in which care is provided and includes resources such as equipment and staffing levels.

    B. **CORRECT:** An outcome audit evaluates the effectiveness of nursing care. It should include observable data such as infection rates among clients.

    C. **CORRECT:** A root cause analysis is indicated when a sentinel event occurs. A sentinel event is a serious problem such as injury to or death of a client. Immediate investigation of the problem is indicated. The health care team may use root cause analysis to study the problem and take measures to prevent reoccurrence.

    D. INCORRECT: Retrospective audits are conducted when the client is no longer receiving care.

    E. **CORRECT:** The benchmark is set at the beginning of the process and then it is compared to the data after collection is completed.

    (N) NCLEX® Connection: Management of Care, Performance Improvement (Quality Improvement)

8. A. INCORRECT: The frequency with which the procedure is performed is important. The team may take the frequency in which the procedure is performed under consideration in the planning process, but this information does not address the efficacy of the procedure.

    B. INCORRECT: The team may take client satisfaction under consideration in the planning process, but this information does not address the efficacy of the procedure.

    C. **CORRECT:** The incidence of complications related to the procedure is an outcome measure related to the efficacy of the procedure.

    D. INCORRECT: The team may take accuracy of documentation under consideration in the planning process, but this information does not address the efficacy of the procedure.

    (N) NCLEX® Connection: Management of Care, Performance Improvement (Quality Improvement)

9. A. **CORRECT:** The goal in resolving conflict is a win-win situation. The unit manager is using an ineffective strategy, avoidance, to deal with this conflict. She is aware of the conflict but is not attempting to resolve it.

    B. INCORRECT: The goal in resolving conflict is a win-win solution. When smoothing is used, one person attempts to "smooth" the other party and/or attempts to point out areas in which the parties agree. This is typically a lose-lose solution.

    C. INCORRECT: The goal in resolving a conflict is a win-win solution. When cooperating is used, one party allows the other party to win. This is a lose-win solution.

    D. INCORRECT: The goal in resolving a conflict is a win-win solution. When negotiating is used, each party gives up something. If one party gives up more than the other, this can become a win-lose solution.

    (N) NCLEX® Connection: Management of Care, Concepts of Management

10. A. INCORRECT: The nurse manager should conduct the evaluation in a private setting such as the unit manger's office.

    B. INCORRECT: The performance appraisal should include information collected from the entire time span of the appraisal.

    C. **CORRECT:** The unit manager should only use data that has been observed and formally documented.

    D. INCORRECT: The nurse should be involved in the appraisal process. It is appropriate to require the nurse to complete a self-appraisal prior to the meeting.

    Ⓝ NCLEX® Connection: Management of Care, Concepts of Management

11. *Using the Active Learning Template: Basic Concept*

    A. Related Content
       • Emotional intelligence is the ability of an individual to perceive and manage the emotions of self and others.

    B. Underlying Principles
       • Insight into the emotions of members of the team.
       • Understands the perspective of others.
       • Encourages constructive criticism and is open to new ideas.
       • Able to maintain focus while multitasking.
       • Manages emotions and channels them in a positive direction, which in turn helps the team accomplish its goals.
       • Committed to the delivery of high-quality client care.
       • Refrains from judgment in controversial or emotionally charged situations until facts are gathered.

    Ⓝ NCLEX® Connection: Management of Care, Concepts of Management

CHAPTER 2 Coordinating Client Care

TOPICS

› Collaboration with the Interdisciplinary Team
› Principles of Case Management
› Continuity of Care: Consultations, Referrals, Transfers, and Discharge Planning

NCLEX® CONNECTIONS

When reviewing the chapters in this unit, keep in mind the relevant sections of the NCLEX® outline, in particular:

Client Needs: Management of Care

› Relevant topics/tasks include:

» Case Management

› Explore resources available to assist the client with achieving or maintaining independence.

» Collaboration with Interdisciplinary Team

› Review the plan of care to ensure continuity across disciplines.

» Concepts of Management

› Act as a liaison between the client and others.

» Consultation

› Use clinical decision making/critical thinking in consultation situations.

» Continuity of Care

› Maintain continuity of care between/among health care agencies.

» Referrals

› Identify community resources for the client.

CHAPTER 2	Coordinating Client Care

Overview

- One of the primary roles of nursing is the coordination and management of client care in collaboration with the health care team.
- In so doing, high-quality health care is provided as clients move through the health care system in a cost-effective and time-efficient manner.
- To effectively coordinate client care, a nurse must have an understanding of:
  - Collaboration With the Interprofessional Team
  - Principles of Case Management
  - Continuity of Care (including consultations, referrals, transfers, and discharge planning)

COLLABORATION WITH THE INTERPROFESSIONAL TEAM

Overview

- An interprofessional team is a group of health care professionals from various disciplines.
- Collaboration involves discussion of client care issues in making health care decisions, especially for clients who have multiple problems. The specialized knowledge and skills of each discipline are used in the development of an interprofessional plan of care that addresses multiple problems. Nurses should recognize that the collaborative efforts of the interprofessional team allow the achievement of results that a team member would be incapable of accomplishing alone.
  - Nurse-provider collaboration should be fostered to create a climate of mutual respect and collaborative practice.
  - Collaboration occurs among different levels of nurses and nurses with different areas of expertise.
  - Collaboration should also occur between the interprofessional team, the client, and the client's family/significant others when an interprofessional plan of care is being developed.
  - Collaboration is a form of conflict resolution that results in a win-win solution for both the client and health care team.

Nursing Role Within the Interprofessional Team

- Qualities needed by the nurse for effective collaboration include the following:
  - Good communication skills
  - Assertiveness
  - Conflict negotiation skills
  - Leadership skills
  - Professional presence
  - Decision making and critical thinking

- The nurse's role is to provide:
  - Coordination of the interprofessional team
  - A holistic understanding of the client, the client's health care needs, and the health care system
  - The opportunity for care to be provided with continuity over time and across disciplines
  - The client with the opportunity to be a partner in the development of the plan of care
  - Information during rounds and interprofessional team meetings regarding the status of the client's health
  - An avenue for the initiation of a consultation related to a specific health care issue
  - A link to postdischarge resources that may need a referral
- Variables that affect collaboration with the interprofessional team
  - Decision-making styles
    - The interprofessional team within a facility is challenged with making sound decisions about how client care is delivered. A variety of decision-making styles are available for use as appropriate. Often the group leader decides the decision-making style the team will use. Decision-making styles vary in regard to the amount of data collected and the number of options generated.
      - Decisive – The team uses a minimum amount of data and generates one option.
      - Flexible – The team uses a limited amount of data and generates several options.
      - Hierarchical – The team uses a large amount of data and generates one option.
      - Integrative – The team uses a large amount of data and generates several options.
  - Hierarchical influence on decision-making
    - Decision-making is also influenced by the facility hierarchy. In a centralized hierarchy, nurses at the top of the organizational chart make most of the decisions. In a decentralized hierarchy, staff nurses who provide direct client care are included in the decision-making process. Large organizations benefit from the use of decentralized decision-making because managers at the top of the hierarchy do not have firsthand knowledge of unit-level challenges or problems. Decentralized decision-making promotes job satisfaction among staff nurses.
  - Behavioral change strategies
    - Although bombarded with constant change, members of the interprofessional team can be resistant to change. Three strategies a manager can use to promote change are the rational-empirical, normative-reeducative and the power-coercive. Often the manager uses a combination of these strategies.
      - Rational-empirical – The manager provides factual information to support the change. Used when resistance to change is minimal.
      - Normative-reeducative – The manager focuses on interpersonal relationships to promote change.
      - Power-coercive – The manger uses rewards to promote change. Used when individuals are highly resistant to change.

○ Stages of team formation

■ Teams typically work through a group formation process before reaching peak performance. The stages of team formation are as follows:

□ Forming – Members of the team get to know each other. The leader defines tasks for the team and offers direction.

□ Storming – Conflict arises, and team members begin to express polarized views. The team establishes rules, and members begin to take on various roles.

□ Norming – The team establishes rules. Members show respect for one another and begin to accomplish some of the tasks.

□ Performing – The team focuses on accomplishment of tasks.

○ Impact of generational differences among members of an interprofessional team

■ Generational differences influence the value system of the members of an interprofessional team and can affect how members function within the team. Generational differences can be challenging for members of a team, but working with individuals from different generations also can bring strength to the team. Characteristics of each generational group are provided below:

GENERATION	APPROXIMATE BIRTH YEAR RANGE	CHARACTERISTICS
Veteran	1925-1942	› Supports the status quo. › Accepts authority. › Appreciates hierarchy. › Loyal to employer.
Baby boomer	1943-1960	› Accepts authority. › Workaholics. › Some struggle with new technology. › Loyal to employer.
Generation X	1961-1980	› Adapts easily to change. › Personal life and family are important. › Proficient with technology. › Makes frequent job changes.
Generation Y	1981-2000	› Optimistic and self-confident. › Values achievement. › Technology is a way of life. › At ease with cultural diversity.

○ Magnet Recognition Program

■ The interprofessional team is charged with maintaining continuous quality improvement. The nursing staff may choose to demonstrate quality nursing care by seeking Magnet Recognition. The American Nurses Credentialing Center awards Magnet Recognition to health care facilities that provide high-quality client care and attract and retain well-qualified nurses. The term magnet is used to recognize the facility's power to draw nurses to the facility and to retain them. Fourteen forces of magnetism provide the framework for the magnet review process. The first step for a facility that applies for magnet recognition is to complete a self-appraisal based on a set of established standards. It is important that all levels of nursing participate in the application process. After documentation that the standards have been met, an on-site appraisal is conducted. A facility that meets the standards is awarded magnet status for a four-year period. To maintain magnet status, the facility must maintain the established standards and submit an annual report.

PRINCIPLES OF CASE MANAGEMENT

Overview

- Case management is the coordination of care provided by an interprofessional team from the time a client starts receiving care until he or she is no longer receiving services.

- Case management focuses on managed care of the client through collaboration of the health care team in both inpatient and postacute settings for insured individuals.

- The goal of case management is to avoid fragmentation of care and control cost.

- A case manager collaborates with the interprofessional health care team during the assessment of a client's needs and subsequent care planning, and follows up by monitoring the achievement of desired client outcomes within established time parameters.

  - A case manager may be a nurse, social worker, or other designated health care professional.

    - A case manager's role and knowledge expectations are extensive; therefore, case managers are required to have advanced practice degrees or advanced training in this area.

  - Case manager nurses do not usually provide direct client care.

  - Case managers usually oversee a caseload of clients with similar disorders or treatment regimens.

  - Case managers in the community coordinate resources and services for clients whose care is based in a residential setting.

- A critical or clinical pathway or care map may be used to support the implementation of clinical guidelines and protocols. These tools are usually based on cost and length of stay parameters mandated by prospective payment systems such as Medicare and insurance companies.

Nursing Role in Case Management

- The nurse's role in case management involves the following:

  - Coordinating care, particularly for clients who have complex health care needs

  - Facilitating continuity of care

  - Improving efficiency of care and utilization of resources

  - Enhancing quality of care provided

  - Limiting unnecessary costs and lengthy stays

  - Advocating for the client and family

CONTINUITY OF CARE: CONSULTATIONS, REFERRALS, TRANSFERS, AND DISCHARGE PLANNING

Overview

- Continuity of care refers to the consistency of care provided as clients move through the health care system. It enhances the quality of client care and facilitates the achievement of positive client outcomes.
- Continuity of care is desired as clients move from one:
  - ○ Level of care to another, such as from the ICU to a medical unit
  - ○ Facility to another, such as from an acute care facility to a skilled facility
  - ○ Unit/department to another, such as from the PACU to the postsurgical unit
- Nurses are responsible for facilitating continuity of care and coordinating care through documentation, reporting, and collaboration.
- A formal, written plan of care enhances coordination of care between nurses, interprofessional team members, and primary care providers.

Nursing Role in Continuity of Care

- The nurse's role as coordinator of care includes the following:
  - ○ Facilitating the continuity of care provided by members of the health care team
  - ○ Acting as a representative of the client and as a liaison when collaborating with the provider and other members of the health care team
    - ▪ When acting as a liaison, the nurse serves in the role of client advocate by protecting the rights of clients and ensuring that client needs are met.
- As the coordinator of care, the nurse is responsible for:
  - ○ Admission, transfer, discharge, and postdischarge orders
  - ○ Initiation, revision, and evaluation of the plan of care
  - ○ Reporting the client's status to other nurses and the provider
  - ○ Coordinating the discharge plan
  - ○ Facilitating referrals and the utilization of community resources

Documentation and Communication

- Documentation to facilitate continuity of care includes the following:
  - ○ Graphic records that illustrate trending of assessment data such as vital signs
  - ○ Flow sheets that reflect routine care completed and other care-related data
  - ○ Nurses' notes that describe changes in client status or unusual circumstances

- Client care summaries that serve as quick references for client care information
- Nursing care plans that set the standard for care provided:
  - Standardized nursing care plans provide a starting point for the nurse responsible for care plan development.
  - Standardized plans must be individualized to each client.
  - All documentation should reflect the plan of care.
- Communication and Continuity of Care
  - Communication Tools
    - Poor communication can lead to adverse outcomes, including sentinel events (unexpected death or serious injury of a client).
    - A number of communication hand-off tools are available for use to improve communication and promote client safety: I-SBAR, PACE, I PASS the BATON, Five P's
  - Change-of-shift report
    - Performed with the nurse who is assuming responsibility for the client's care.
    - Describes the current health status of the client.
    - Informs the next shift of pertinent client care information.
    - Provides the oncoming nurse the opportunity to ask questions and clarify the plan of care.
    - Should be given in a private area, such as a conference room or at the bedside, to protect client confidentiality.
  - Reports to the provider
    - Assessment data integral to changes in client status
    - Recommendations for changes in the plan of care
    - Clarification of orders

Consultations

- A consultant is a professional who provides expert advice in a particular area. A consultation is requested to help determine what treatment/services the client requires.
- Consultants provide expertise for clients who require a specific type of knowledge or service (a cardiologist for a client who had a myocardial infarction, a psychiatrist for a client whose risk for suicide must be assessed).
- The nurse's role with regard to consultations is to:
  - Initiate the necessary consults or notify the provider of the client's needs so the consult can be initiated.
  - Provide the consultant with all pertinent information about the problem (information from the client/family, the client's medical records).
  - Incorporate the consultant's recommendations into the client's plan of care.

Referrals

- A referral is a formal request for a special service by another care provider. It is made so that the client can access the care identified by the provider or the consultant.
- The care may be provided in the inpatient setting or outside the facility.
- Clients being discharged from health care facilities to their home may still require nursing care.
- Discharge referrals are based on client needs in relation to actual and potential problems and may be facilitated with the assistance of social services, especially if there is a need for:
  ○ Specialized equipment (cane, walker, wheelchair, grab bars in bathroom)
  ○ Specialized therapists (physical, occupational, speech)
  ○ Care providers (home health nurse, hospice nurse, home health aide)
- Knowledge of community and online resources is necessary to appropriately link the client with needed services.
- The nurse's role with regard to referrals is to:
  ○ Begin discharge planning upon the client's admission.
  ○ Evaluate client/family competencies in relation to home care prior to discharge.
  ○ Involve the client and family in care planning.
  ○ Collaborate with other health care professionals to ensure all health care needs are met and necessary referrals are made.
  ○ Complete referral forms to ensure proper reimbursement for prescribed services.

Transfers

- Clients may be transferred from one unit to another, one department to another, or one facility to another.
- Continuity of care must be maintained as the client moves from one setting to another.

- The use of communication hand-off tools (I PASS the BATON, PACE) promotes continuity of care and client safety.
- The nurse's role in regard to transfers is to provide a written and verbal report of the client's status and care needs including:
  ○ Client medical diagnosis and care providers
  ○ Client demographic information
  ○ Overview of client's health status, plan of care, and recent progress
  ○ Any alterations that may precipitate an immediate concern
  ○ Most recent set of vital signs and medications, including when a PRN was given
  ○ Notification of any assessments or client care that will be needed within the next few hours
  ○ Allergies
  ○ Diet and activity prescriptions

- ○ Presence of or need for special equipment or adaptive devices (oxygen, suction, wheelchair)
- ○ Advance directives and whether the client is to be resuscitated in the event of cardiac or respiratory arrest
- ○ Family involvement in care and health care proxy, if applicable

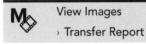

View Images

› Transfer Report   › Interfacility Transfer Form

Discharge Planning

- Discharge planning is an interprofessional process that is started by the nurse at the time of the client's admission.
  - ○ The nurse conducts discharge planning with both the client and client's family for optimal results.
  - ○ Discharge planning serves as a starting point for continuity of care. As client care needs are identified, measures can be taken to prepare for the provision of needed support.
  - ○ The need for additional services such as home health, outpatient therapy, and respite care can be addressed before the client is discharged so the service is in place when the client arrives home.
- A client who leaves a facility without orders from the provider is considered leaving "against medical advice," or AMA. A client who is legally competent has the legal right to leave the facility at any time. The nurse should immediately notify the provider. If the client is at risk for harm, it is also imperative that the nurse explain the risk involved in leaving the facility. A form should be signed by the individual relinquishing responsibility for any complications that arise from discontinuing prescribed care. The nurse should document all communication, as well as the specific advice that was provided for the client. A nurse who tries to prevent the client from leaving the facility may face legal charges of assault, battery, and false imprisonment.
- Discharge instructions should include the following:
  - ○ Step-by-step instructions for procedures to be done at home
    - Clients should be given the opportunity to provide a return demonstration of these procedures to validate learning.
  - ○ Medication regimen instructions for home, including adverse effects and actions to take to minimize them.
  - ○ Precautions to take when performing procedures or administering medications
  - ○ Indications of medication adverse effects or medical complications that should be reported to the provider
  - ○ Names and numbers of health care providers and community services the client/family can contact
  - ○ Plans for follow-up care and therapies

- The nurse's role with regard to discharge is to provide a written summary including:
  - ○ Type of discharge (ordered by provider, AMA)
  - ○ Date and time of discharge, who accompanied the client, and how the client was transported (wheelchair to a private car, stretcher to an ambulance)
  - ○ Discharge destination (home, long-term care facility)
  - ○ A summary of the client's condition at discharge (gait, dietary intake, use of assistive devices, blood glucose)
  - ○ A description of any unresolved problems and plans for follow-up
  - ○ Disposition of valuables, client's medications brought from home, and/or prescriptions
  - ○ A copy of the client's discharge instructions

 View Image: Discharge Summary

APPLICATION EXERCISES

1. A nurse is preparing to transfer an older adult client who is 72 hr postoperative from a surgical procedure to a long-term care facility. Which of the following should the nurse include in the transfer report? (Select all that apply).

_____ A. Type of anesthesia used

_____ B. The client's advance directives status

_____ C. The client's vital signs on day of admission

_____ D. The client's medical diagnosis

_____ E. Need for special equipment

2. A nurse is participating in an interprofessional conference for a client who has a recent C6 spinal cord injury. The client worked as a construction worker prior to his injury. Which of the following members of the interprofessional team should also participate in planning care for this client? (Select all that apply.)

_____ A. Physical therapist

_____ B. Speech therapist

_____ C. Occupational therapist

_____ D. Psychologist

_____ E. Vocational counselor

3. A nurse manager is working with a committee of nurses whose task is to update the policies for new employee orientation. The nurse manager directs the team to collect as much data as possible and recommend several options. Which of the following decision-making styles is being demonstrated by the nurse manager?

A. Decisive

B. Flexible

C. Hierarchical

D Integrative

4. A nurse who has just assumed the role of unit manger is examining her skills in interprofessional collaboration. Which of the following actions support interprofessional collaboration? (Select all that apply.)

_____ A. Use aggressive communication when addressing the team.

_____ B. Recognize the knowledge and skills of each member of the team.

_____ C. Ensure that a nurse is assigned to serve as the group facilitator for all interdisciplinary meetings.

_____ D. Encourage the client and family to participate in the team meeting.

_____ E. Support team member requests for referral.

5. A nurse on a telemetry unit is caring for a client who was admitted 2 hr ago and has chest pain. The client becomes angry and tells the nurse that there is nothing wrong with him and that he is going home immediately. The nurse should base her actions on which of the following? (Select all that apply.)

_____ A. The nurse should notify the risk manager immediately.

_____ B. In the event the client leaves the hospital without a discharge order, the nurse should document that the client left the facility "against medical advice" (AMA).

_____ C. It is the nurse's responsibility to explain to the client the risks involved if he chooses to leave.

_____ D. Most facilities have a form that clients are asked to sign if they leave the facility prior to discharge.

_____ E. A nurse who tries to prevent a client from leaving the hospital may be faced with legal charges.

6. A nurse is explaining her role as case manager to her preceptor. What should the case manager include in her discussion? Use the ATI Active Learning Template: Basic Concept to complete this item. Identify three roles of a case manager.

APPLICATION EXERCISES KEY

1. A. INCORRECT: The nurse should include only information that is pertinent in the transfer report.

    B. **CORRECT:** The nurse should include information that is pertinent and that the next nurse will need when providing care.

    C. INCORRECT: The nurse should include only information that is pertinent in the transfer report. The nurse should include the client's most recent vital signs.

    D. **CORRECT:** The nurse should include information that is pertinent and that the next nurse will need when providing care.

    E. **CORRECT:** The nurse should include information that is pertinent and that the next nurse will need when providing care.

    (N) NCLEX® Connection: Management of Care, Continuity of Care

2. A. **CORRECT:** The client will need the assistance of a physical therapist to assist will mobility skills and to maintain muscle strength.

    B. INCORRECT: A speech therapist assists a client who has speech and swallowing problems, which are not anticipated for this client.

    C. **CORRECT:** The client will need the assistance of an occupational therapist to learn how to perform the activities of daily living.

    D. **CORRECT:** The client will need the assistance of a psychologist to adapt to the psychosocial impact of the injury.

    E. **CORRECT:** The client will need the assistance of a vocational counselor to explore options for reemployment.

    (N) NCLEX® Connection: Management of Care, Collaboration with Interdisciplinary Team

3. A. INCORRECT: When the decisive decision-making style is used, the team uses a minimum amount of data and generates one option.

    B. INCORRECT: When the flexible decision-making style is used, the team uses a limited amount of data and generates several options.

    C. INCORRECT: When the hierarchical decision-making style is used,the team uses a large amount of data and generates one option.

    D. **CORRECT:** When the integrative decision-making style is used, the team uses a large amount of data and generates several options.

    (N) NCLEX® Connection: Management of Care, Concepts of Management

4. A. INCORRECT: The nurse should use assertive skills when communicating with the interprofessional team.

   B. **CORRECT:** The nurse should recognize that each member of the team has specific skills to assist the client with rehabilitation.

   C. INCORRECT: A nurse can serve as the facilitator, but this role can be assumed by any member of the team.

   D. **CORRECT:** Collaboration should occur among the client, family, and interprofessional team.

   E. **CORRECT:** The nurse should support suggestions for referrals to link clients to appropriate resources.

   (N) NCLEX® Connection: Management of Care, Collaboration with Interdisciplinary Team

5. A. INCORRECT: The nurse does not need to notify the risk manager immediately. However, it is imperative that the nurse notify the provider of the client's intention to leave so the provider can intervene and decrease the risk of a negative client outcome.

   B. **CORRECT:** When documenting a client's discharge, the nurse should document the type of discharge, including an AMA discharge.

   C. **CORRECT:** If the client leaves before the provider arrives, the nurse is legally responsible to warn the client of the risks involved in leaving the hospital.

   D. **CORRECT:** Clients who leave the hospital prior to discharge are asked to sign a form to provide legal protection for the hospital.

   E. **CORRECT:** A nurse who tries to prevent a client from leaving the hospital by any action, such as threatening him, or refusing to give him his clothes, may be charged with assault, battery, and false imprisonment.

   (N) NCLEX® Connection: Management of Care, Client Rights

6. *Using ATI Active Learning Template: Basic Concept*
   - Roles of a Case Manager
     - Coordinating care of clients who have complex health care needs
     - Facilitating continuity of care
     - Improving efficiency of care
     - Enhancing quality of care provided
     - Limiting cost and lengthy stays
     - Advocating for the client and family

   (N) NCLEX® Connection: Management of Care, Concepts of Management

CHAPTER 3 Professional Responsibilities

TOPICS

› Client Rights
› Advocacy
› Informed Consent
› Advance Directives
› Confidentiality and Information Security
› Legal Practice
› Disruptive Behavior
› Ethical Practice

NCLEX® CONNECTIONS

When reviewing the chapters in this unit, keep in mind the relevant sections of the NCLEX® outline, in particular:

Client Needs: Management of Care

› Relevant topics/tasks include:
  » Advance Directives
    › Integrate advance directives into the client's plan of care.
  » Advocacy
    › Discuss identified treatment options with clients and respect their decisions.
  » Client Rights
    › Educate clients and staff about client rights and responsibilities.
  » Confidentiality/Information Security
    › Assess staff member and client understanding of confidentiality requirements.
  » Ethical Practice
    › Recognize ethical dilemmas and take appropriate action.
  » Information Technology
    › Use emerging technology in managing client health care.
  » Informed Consent
    › Verify that the client comprehends and consents to care/procedures, including procedures requiring informed consent.
  » Legal Rights and Responsibilities
    › Educate the client/staff on legal issues.

Overview

- Professional responsibilities are the obligations that nurses have to their clients.
- To meet their professional responsibilities, nurses must be knowledgeable in the following areas:
  - Client Rights
  - Advocacy
  - Informed Consent
  - Advance Directives
  - Confidentiality and Information Security
  - Legal Practice
  - Disruptive Behavior
  - Ethical Practice

CLIENT RIGHTS

Overview

- Client rights are the legal guarantees that clients have with regard to their health care.
  - Clients using the services of a health care institution retain their rights as individuals and citizens of the United States. The American Hospital Association (AHA) identifies client rights in health care settings in "The Patient Care Partnership." For more information regarding this document, go to www.aha.org.
  - Residents in nursing facilities that participate in Medicare programs similarly retain "Resident Rights" under statutes that govern the operation of these facilities.
- Nurses are accountable for protecting the rights of clients. Situations that require particular attention include informed consent, refusal of treatment, advance directives, confidentiality, and information security.

Nursing Role in Client Rights

- Nurses must ensure that clients understand their rights, and nurses also must protect clients' rights during nursing care.
- Regardless of the client's age, the client's nursing needs, or the setting in which care is provided, the basic tenants are the same. Each client has the right to:
  - Be informed about all aspects of care and take an active role in the decision-making process.
  - Accept, refuse, or request modification to the plan of care.
  - Receive care that is delivered by competent individuals who treat the client with respect.

- Refusal of Treatment
  - The Patient Self-Determination Act (PSDA) stipulates that on admission to a health care facility, all clients must be informed of their right to accept or refuse care. Competent adults have the right to refuse treatment, including the right to leave a health care facility without a discharge order from the provider.
  - If the client refuses a treatment or procedure, the client is asked to sign a document indicating that he understands the risk involved with refusing the treatment or procedure, and that he has chosen to refuse it.
  - When a client decides to leave the facility without a discharge order, the nurse notifies the provider and discusses with the client the potential risks associated with leaving the facility prior to discharge.
  - The nurse carefully documents the information that was provided to the client and that notification of the provider occurred. The client should be informed of the following:
    - Possible complications that could occur without treatment.
    - Possibility of permanent physical or mental impairment or disability.
    - Possibility of other complications that could lead to death.
  - The client is asked to sign an "Against Medical Advice" form.
  - If the client refuses to sign the form, this is also documented by the nurse.

 View Video: Client Rights

ADVOCACY

Overview

- Advocacy refers to nurses' role in supporting clients by ensuring that they are properly informed, that their rights are respected, and that they are receiving the proper level of care.
- Advocacy is one of the most important roles of the nurse, especially when clients are unable to speak or act for themselves.
- As an advocate, the nurse ensures that the client has the information he needs to make decisions about health care.
- Nurses must act as advocates even when they disagree with clients' decisions.
- The complex health care system puts clients in a vulnerable position, and nurses are their voice when the system is not acting in their best interest.
- The nursing profession also has a responsibility to support and advocate for legislation that promotes public policies that protect clients as consumers and create a safe environment for their care.

Nursing Role in Advocacy

- As advocates, nurses must ensure that clients are informed of their rights and have adequate information on which to base health care decisions.

- Nurses must be careful to assist clients with making health care decisions and not direct or control their decisions.

- Nurses may need to mediate on the client's behalf when the actions of others are not in the client's best interest or changes need to be made in the plan of care.

- Situations in which nurses may need to advocate for clients or assist them to advocate for themselves include:

  ○ End-of-life decisions

  ○ Access to health care

  ○ Protection of client privacy

  ○ Informed consent

  ○ Substandard practice

- Nurses are accountable for their actions even if they are carrying out a provider's prescription. It is the nurse's responsibility to question a provider's prescription if it could harm a client (incorrect dosage for a medication, potential adverse interaction with another prescribed medication, contraindication due to a client allergy or medical history).

ESSENTIAL COMPONENTS OF ADVOCACY			
Skills		Values	
› Risk-taking	› Articulate communication	› Caring	› Respect
› Vision		› Autonomy	› Empowerment
› Self-confidence	› Assertiveness		

   View Video: Client Advocacy

INFORMED CONSENT

Overview

- Informed consent is a legal process by which a client has given written permission for a procedure or treatment to be performed. Consent is considered to be informed when the client has been provided with and understands:

  - The reason the treatment or procedure is needed

  - How the treatment or procedure will benefit the client

  - The risks involved if the client chooses to receive treatment or procedure

  - Other options to treat the problem, including the option of not treating the problem

  - The risk involved if the client chooses no treatment

- The nurse's role in the informed consent process is to witness the client's signature on the informed consent form and to ensure that informed consent has been appropriately obtained.

- The nurse should seek the assistance of an interpreter if the client does not speak and understand the language used by the provider.

Informed Consent Guidelines

- Consent is required for all care given in a health care facility. For most aspects of nursing care, implied consent is adequate. The client provides implied consent when she complies with the instructions provided by the nurse. For example, the nurse is preparing to administer a TB skin test, and the client holds out her arm for the nurse.

- For an invasive procedure or surgery, the client is required to provide written consent.

- State laws regulate who is able to give informed consent. Laws vary regarding age limitations and emergencies. Nurses are responsible for knowing the laws in the state of practice.

- Signing an informed consent form

  - The form for informed consent must be signed by a competent adult.

  - The person who signs the form must be capable of understanding the information provided by the health care professional who will be providing the service, and the person must be able to fully communicate in return with the health care professional.

  - When the person giving the informed consent is unable to communicate due to a language barrier or hearing impairment, a trained medical interpreter must be provided. Many health care agencies contract with professional interpreters who have additional skills in medical terminology to assist with providing information.

- Individuals authorized to grant consent for another person include:

  - Parent of a minor

  - Legal guardian

  - Court-specified representative

  - Spouse or closest available individual who has durable power of attorney for health care

- Emancipated minors (minors who are independent from their parents, such as a married minor) can provide informed consent for themselves.
- The nurse must verify that consent is informed and witness the client sign the consent form.

RESPONSIBILITIES FOR INFORMED CONSENT		
The Provider	The Client	The Nurse
› Obtains informed consent. To do so, the provider must give the client: » A complete description of the treatment/procedure » A description of the professionals who will be performing and participating in the treatment » A description of the potential harm, pain, and/or discomfort that might occur » Options for other treatments » The right to refuse treatment » The risk involved if the client chooses no treatment	› Gives informed consent. To give informed consent, the client must: » Give it voluntarily (no coercion involved). » Be competent and of legal age or be an emancipated minor. (If the client is unable to provide consent, an authorized person must give consent). » Receive sufficient information to make a decision based on an informed understanding of what is expected.	› Witnesses informed consent. The nurse is responsible for: » Ensuring that the provider gave the client the necessary information » Ensuring that the client understood the information and is competent to give informed consent » Having the client sign the informed consent document » Notifying the provider if the client has more questions or does not understand any of the information provided. (The provider is then responsible for giving clarification.) › Documenting: » Reinforcement of information originally given by the provider » That questions the client had were forwarded to the provider » Use of an interpreter

ADVANCE DIRECTIVES

Overview

- The purpose of advance directives is to communicate a client's wishes regarding end-of-life care should the client become unable to do so.
- The Patient Self-Determination Act (PSDA) requires that all clients admitted to a health care facility be asked if they have advance directives.
  - A client without advance directives must be given written information that outlines her rights related to health care decisions and how to formulate advance directives.
  - A health care representative should be available to help with this process.
- Two components of an advance directive are the living will and the durable power of attorney for health care.

Components of Advance Directives

- Living Will

  - A living will is a legal document that expresses the client's wishes regarding medical treatment in the event the client becomes incapacitated and is facing end-of-life issues. Types of treatments that are often addressed in a living will are those that have the capacity to prolong life. Examples of treatments that are addressed are cardiopulmonary resuscitation, mechanical ventilation, and feeding by artificial means.

  - Living wills are legal in all states. However, state statutes and individual health care facility policies may vary. Nurses need to be familiar with their state statute and facility policies.

  - Most state laws include provisions that health care providers who follow the health care directive in a living will are protected from liability.

 View Image: Advance Directives

- Durable Power of Attorney for Health Care

  - A durable power of attorney for health care is a legal document that designates a health care proxy, who is an individual authorized to make health care decisions for a client who is unable. The person who serves in the role of health care proxy to make decisions for the client should be very familiar with the client's wishes. Living wills may be difficult to interpret, especially in the face of unexpected circumstances. A durable power of attorney for health care, as an adjunct to a living will, may be a more effective way of ensuring that the client's decisions about health care are honored.

- Provider's Orders

  - Unless a do not resuscitate (DNR) or allow natural death (AND) order is written, the nurse should initiate CPR when a client has no pulse or respirations. The written order for a DNR or AND must be placed in the client's medical record. The provider consults the client and the family prior to administering a DNR or AND.

  - Additional orders by the provider are based on the client's individual needs and decisions and provide for comfort measures. The client's decision is respected in regard to the use of antibiotics, initiation of diagnostic tests, and provision of nutrition by artificial means.

Nursing Role in Advance Directives

- Nursing responsibilities regarding advance directives include:

  - Providing written information regarding advance directives

  - Documenting the client's advance directives status

  - Ensuring that advance directives are current and reflective of the client's current decisions

  - Recognizing that the client's choice takes priority when there is a conflict between the client and family, or between the client and the provider

  - Informing all members of the health care team of the client's advance directives

CONFIDENTIALITY AND INFORMATION SECURITY

Overview

- Clients have the right to privacy and confidentiality in relation to their health care information and medical recommendations.

- Nurses who disclose client information to an unauthorized person can be liable for invasion of privacy, defamation, or slander.

- The security and privacy rules of the Health Insurance Portability and Accountability Act (HIPAA) were enacted to protect the confidentiality of health care information and to give the client the right to control the release of information. Specific rights provided by the legislation includes the following:

  - The rights of clients to obtain a copy of their medical record and to submit requests to amend erroneous or incomplete information

  - A requirement for health care providers and insurance providers to provide written information about how medical information is used and how it is shared with other entities (permission must be obtained before information is shared)

  - The rights of clients to privacy and confidentiality

Nursing Role in Confidentiality

- It is essential for nurses to be aware of the rights of clients in regard to privacy and confidentiality. Facility policies and procedures are established in order to ensure compliance with HIPAA regulations. It is essential that nurses know and adhere to the policies and procedures. HIPAA regulations also provide for penalties in the event of noncompliance with the regulations.

- The Privacy Rule of HIPAA requires that nurses protect all written and verbal communication about clients. Components of the privacy rule include:

  - Only health care team members directly responsible for the client's care should be allowed access to the client's records. Nurses may not share information with other clients or staff not involved in the care of the client.

  - Clients have a right to read and obtain a copy of their medical record, and agency policy should be followed when the client requests to read or have a copy of the record.

  - No part of the client record can be copied except for authorized exchange of documents between health care institutions. For example:

    - Transfer from a hospital to an extended care facility

    - Exchange of documents between a general practitioner and a specialist during a consult

  - Client medical records must be kept in a secure area to prevent inappropriate access to the information. Using public display boards to list client names and diagnoses is restricted.

  - Electronic records should be password-protected, and care must be taken to prevent public viewing of the information.

    - Health care workers should use only their own passwords to access information.

- ○ Client information may not be disclosed to unauthorized individuals, including family members who request it and individuals who call on the phone.
  - Many hospitals use a code system in which information is only disclosed to individuals who can provide the code.
  - Nurses should ask any individual inquiring about a client's status for the code and disclose information only when an individual can give the code.
- ○ Communication about a client should only take place in a private setting where it cannot be overheard by unauthorized individuals. The practice of "walking rounds," where other clients and visitors can hear what is being said, is no longer sanctioned. Taped rounds also are discouraged because nurses should not receive information about clients for whom they are not responsible. Change-of-shift reports can be done at the bedside as long as the client does not have a roommate and no unsolicited visitors are present.

- Information Security
  - ○ Health information systems (HIS) are used to manage administrative functions and clinical functions. The clinical portion of the system is often referred to as the clinical information systems (CIS). The CIS may be used to coordinate essential aspects of client care.
  - ○ In order to comply with HIPAA regulations, each health care facility has specific policies and procedures designed to monitor staff adherence, technical protocols, computer privacy, and data safety.
  - ○ Information security protocols include:
    - Logging off from the computer before leaving the workstation to ensure that others cannot view protected health information (PHI) on the monitor
    - Never sharing a user ID or password with anyone
    - Never leaving a client's chart or other printed or written PHI where others can access it
    - Shredding any printed or written client information used for reporting or client care after it is no longer needed

- Use of Social Media
  - ○ The use of social media by members of the nursing profession is common practice. The benefits to using social media are numerous. It provides a mechanism for nurses to access current information about health care and enhances communication among nurses, colleagues, and clients and families. It also provides an opportunity for nurses to express concerns and seek support from others. But nurses must be cautious about the risk of intentional or inadvertent breaches of confidentiality via social media.
  - ○ The right to privacy is a fundamental component of client care. Invasion of privacy as it relates to health care is the release of client health information to others without the client's consent. Confidentiality is the duty of the nurse to protect a client's private information.
  - ○ The inappropriate use of social media can result in a breach of client confidentiality. Depending on the circumstances, the consequences can include termination of employment by the employer, discipline by the board of nursing, charges of defamation or invasion of privacy, and in the most serious of circumstances, federal charges for violation of the Health Insurance Portability and Accountability Act (HIPAA).
  - ○ Protecting Yourself and Others
    - Become familiar with facility policies about the use of social media, and adhere to them.
    - Avoid disclosing any client health information online. Be sure no one can overhear conversations about a client when speaking on the telephone.

- Do not take or share photos or videos of a client.

- Remember to maintain professional boundaries when interacting with clients online.

- Never post a belittling or offensive remark about a client, employer, or coworker.

- Report any violations of facility social media policies to the nurse manager.

LEGAL PRACTICE

 Overview

- In order to be safe practitioners, nurses must understand the legal aspects of the nursing profession.

- Understanding the laws governing nursing practice allows nurses to protect client rights and to reduce the risk of nursing liability.

- Nurses are accountable for practicing nursing in accordance with the various sources of law affecting nursing practice. It is important that nurses know and comply with these laws. By practicing nursing within the confines of the law, nurses are able to:

  ○ Provide safe competent care.

  ○ Advocate for clients' rights.

  ○ Provide care that is within the nurse's scope of practice.

  ○ Discern the responsibilities of nursing in relation to the responsibilities of other members of the health care team.

  ○ Provide care that is consistent with established standards of care.

  ○ Shield oneself from liability.

Sources of Law

- Federal Regulations

  ○ Federal regulations have a great impact on nursing practice. Some of the federal laws impacting nursing practice include:

    - The Health Insurance Portability and Accountability Act (HIPAA)

    - The Americans with Disabilities Act (ADA)

    - The Mental Health Parity Act (MHPA)

    - The Patient Self-Determination Act (PSDA)

    - The Uniform Anatomical Gift Act and the National Organ Transplant Act

- Criminal and Civil Laws

  ○ Criminal law is a subsection of public law and relates to the relationship of an individual with the government. Violations of criminal law may be categorized as either a felony (a serious crime, such as homicide) or misdemeanor (a less serious crime, such as petty theft). A nurse who falsifies a record to cover up a serious mistake may be found guilty of breaking a criminal law.

○ Civil laws protect the individual rights of people. One type of civil law that relates to the provision of nursing care is tort law. Torts may be classified as unintentional, quasi-intentional, or intentional. Negligence and malpractice (professional negligence) are unintentional torts.

UNINTENTIONAL TORTS	EXAMPLE
Negligence	› A nurse fails to implement safety measures for a client who has been identified as at risk for falls.
Malpractice (professional negligence)	› A nurse administers a large dose of medication due to a calculation error. The client has a cardiac arrest and dies.
QUASI-INTENTIONAL TORTS	**EXAMPLE**
Breach of confidentiality	› A nurse releases the medical diagnosis of a client to a member of the press.
Defamation of character	› A nurse tells a coworker that she believes a client has been unfaithful to the spouse.
INTENTIONAL TORTS	**EXAMPLE**
Assault	› The conduct of one person makes another person fearful and apprehensive (threatening to place a nasogastric tube in a client who is refusing to eat).
Battery	› Intentional and wrongful physical contact with a person that involves an injury or offensive contact (restraining a client and administering an injection against his wishes).
False imprisonment	› A person is confined or restrained against his will (using restraints on a competent client to prevent his leaving the health care facility).

- State Laws
    - The core of nursing practice is regulated by state law.
    - Each state has enacted statutes that define the parameters of nursing practice and give the authority to regulate the practice of nursing to its state board of nursing.
        - Boards of nursing have the authority to adopt rules and regulations that further regulate nursing practice. Although the practice of nursing is similar among states, it is critical that nurses know the laws and rules governing nursing in the state in which they practice.
        - The laws and rules governing nursing practice in a specific state may be accessed at the state board's Web site.
        - Boards of nursing have the authority to both issue and revoke a nursing license.
        - Boards may revoke or suspend a nurse's license for a number of offenses, including practicing without a valid license, habitual use of drugs or alcohol, conviction of a felony, professional negligence, and providing care beyond the scope of practice. Nurses should review the practice act in their states.
        - Boards also set standards for nursing programs and further delineate the scope of practice for registered nurses, licensed practical nurses, and advanced practice nurses.

- ○ Good Samaritan laws, which vary from state to state, protect nurses who provide emergency assistance outside of the employment location. The nurse must provide a standard of care that is reasonable and prudent.

- ○ State laws vary as to when an individual may begin practicing nursing. Some states allow graduates of nursing programs to practice under a limited license, whereas some states require licensure by passing the NCLEX® before working.

- Licensure

  - ○ Until the year 2000, nurses were required to hold a current license in every state in which they practiced. This became problematic with the increase in the electronic practice of nursing. For example, a nurse in one state interprets the reading of a cardiac monitor and provides intervention for a client who is physically located in another state. Additionally, many nurses cross state lines to provide direct care. For example, a nurse who is located near a state border makes home visits on both sides of the state line.

  - ○ To address these issues, the mutual recognition model of nurse licensure (the nurse licensure compact) has been adopted by many states. This model allows nurses who reside in a compact state to practice in another compact state. Nurses must practice in accordance with the statues and rules of the state in which the care is provided. State boards may prohibit a nurse from practicing under the compact if the license of the nurse has been restricted by a board of nursing.

  - ○ Nurses who do not reside in a compact state must practice under the state-based practice model. In other words, if a nurse resides in a non-compact state, the nurse must maintain a current license in every state in which she practices. Some states now require background checks with licensure renewal. It is illegal to practice nursing with an expired license.

Standards of Care (Practice)

- Nurses base practice on established standards of care or legal guidelines for care. These standards of care can be found in:

  - ○ The nurse practice act of each state

    - These acts govern nursing practice, and legal guidelines for practice are established and enforced through a state board of nursing or other government agency.

    - Nurse practice acts vary from state to state, making it obligatory for the nurse to be informed about her state's nurse practice act as it defines the legal parameters of practice.

  - ○ Published standards of nursing practice

    - These are developed by professional organizations such as the American Nurses Association (ANA), the National Association of Practical Nurse Education and Services, Inc. (NAPNES), and speciality organizations such as the American Association of Critical Care Nurses (AACN), the Wound, Ostomy and Continence Nurses Society (WOCN), and the Oncology Nurses Society (ONS).

  - ○ Health care facility policies and procedures

    - Policies and procedures, maintained in the facility's policy and procedure manual, establish the standard of practice for employees of that institution.

    - These manuals provide detailed information about how the nurse should respond to or provide care in specific situations and while performing client care procedures.

- Nurses who practice according to institutional policy are legally protected if that standard of care still results in an injury.
  - If, for example, a client files a complaint with the board of nursing or seeks legal counsel, the nurse who has followed the facility's policies will not usually be charged with misconduct.
- It is very important that nurses are familiar with their institution's policies and procedures and provide client care in accordance with these policies. For example:
  - Assess and document client findings postoperatively according to institutional policy.
  - Change IV tubing and flush saline locks according to institutional policy.

- Standards of care guide, define, and direct the level of care that should be given by practicing nurses. They also are used in malpractice lawsuits to determine if that level was maintained.
- Nurses should refuse to practice beyond the legal scope of practice and/or outside of their areas of competence regardless of reason (staffing shortage, lack of appropriate personnel).
- Nurses should use the formal chain of command to verbalize concerns related to assignment in light of current legal scope of practice, job description, and area of competence.

Professional Negligence

- Professional negligence is the failure of a person with professional training to act in a reasonable and prudent manner. The terms "reasonable and prudent" are generally used to describe a person who has the average judgment, foresight, intelligence, and skill that would be expected of a person with similar training and experience.
- Negligence issues that prompt most malpractice suits include failure to:
  - Follow either professional or facility established standards of care.
  - Use equipment in a responsible and knowledgeable manner.
  - Communicate effectively and thoroughly with the client.
  - Document care that was provided.

THE FIVE ELEMENTS NECESSARY TO PROVE NEGLIGENCE		
Element of Liability	Explanation	Example: Client Who is a Fall Risk
1. Duty to provide care as defined by a standard	› Care that should be given or what a reasonably prudent nurse would do	› The nurse should complete a fall risk assessment for all clients upon admission, per facility protocol.
2. Breach of duty by failure to meet standard	› Failure to give the standard of care that should have been given	› The nurse does not perform a fall risk assessment during admission.
3. Foreseeability of harm	› Knowledge that failing to give the proper standard of care may cause harm to the client	› The nurse should know that failure to take fall-risk precautions may endanger a client at risk for falls.
4. Breach of duty has potential to cause harm (combines elements 2 and 3)	› Failure to meet the standard had potential to cause harm – relationship must be provable	› If a fall risk assessment is not performed, the client's risk for falls is not determined and the proper precautions are not put in place.
5. Harm occurs	› The occurrence of actual harm to the client	› The client falls out of bed and breaks his hip.

- Nurses can avoid being liable for negligence by:
  - Following standards of care
  - Giving competent care
  - Communicating with other health team members
  - Developing a caring rapport with clients
  - Fully documenting assessments, interventions, and evaluations

Impaired Coworkers

- Impaired health care providers pose a significant risk to client safety.

- A nurse who suspects a coworker of using alcohol or drugs while working has a duty to report the coworker to appropriate management personnel as specified by institutional policy. At the time of the infraction, the report may need to be made to the immediate supervisor, such as the charge nurse, to ensure client safety.

- Health care facility policies should provide guidelines for handling employees who have a chemical dependency issue, and many provide peer assistance programs that facilitate the health care provider's entry into a treatment program.

- Each state board of nursing has laws and regulations that govern the disposition of nurses who have been reported secondary to chemical dependency. Depending on the individual case, the boards may have the option to require the nurse to enter a treatment program, during which time the nurse's license may be retained, suspended, or revoked. If a nurse is allowed to maintain licensure, there usually are work restrictions put in place, such as working in noncritical care areas and being restricted from administering controlled medications.

- Health care providers who are found guilty of misappropriation of controlled substances also can be charged with a criminal offense consistent with the infraction.

- Behaviors consistent with chemical dependency that should be considered suspicious include:
  - Smell of alcohol on breath or frequent use of strong mouthwash or mints
  - Impaired coordination, sleepiness, shakiness, and/or slurred speech
  - Bloodshot eyes
  - Mood swings and memory loss
  - Neglect of personal appearance
  - Excessive use of sick leave, tardiness, or absences after a weekend off, holiday, or payday
  - Frequent requests to leave the unit for short periods of time or to leave the shift early
  - Frequently "forgetting" to have another nurse witness wasting of a controlled substance
  - Frequent involvement in incidences where a client assigned to the nurse reports not receiving pain medication or adequate pain relief (impaired nurse provides questionable explanations)
  - Documenting administration of pain medication to a client who did not receive it or documenting a higher dosage than has been given by other nurses
  - Preferring to work the night shift where supervision is less or on units where controlled substances are more frequently given

- Behaviors may be difficult to detect if the impaired nurse is experienced at masking the addiction.

Mandatory Reporting

- In certain situations, health care providers have a legal obligation to report their findings in accordance with state law.
- Abuse
  - All 51 jurisdictions (the 50 states and the District of Colombia) have statutes requiring report of suspicion of child abuse. The statutes set out which occupations are mandatory reporters. In many states, nurses are mandatory reporters.
  - A number of states also mandate that health care providers, including nurses, report suspected abuse of the older adults and dependent adults.
  - Nurses are mandated to report any suspicion of abuse following facility policy.
- Communicable Diseases
  - Nurses are also mandated to report to the proper agency (local health department, state health department) when a client has been diagnosed with a communicable disease.
  - A complete list of reportable diseases and a description of the reporting system are available through the Centers for Disease Control and Prevention Web site, www.cdc.gov. Each state mandates which diseases must be reported in that state. There are more than 60 communicable diseases that must be reported to public health departments to allow officials to:
    - Ensure appropriate medical treatment of diseases (tuberculosis).
    - Monitor for common-source outbreaks (foodborne – hepatitis A).
    - Plan and evaluate control and prevention plans (immunizations for preventable diseases).
    - Identify outbreaks and epidemics.
    - Determine public health priorities based on trends.
    - Educate the community on prevention and treatment of these diseases.

Organ Donation

- Organ and tissue donation is regulated by federal and state laws. Health care facilities have policies and procedures to guide health care workers involved with organ donation.
- Donations may be stipulated in a will or designated on an official card.
- Federal law requires health care facilities to provide access to trained specialists who make the request to clients and/or family members and provide information regarding consent, organ and tissues that can be donated, and how burial or cremation will be impacted by donation.
- Nurses are responsible for answering questions regarding the donation process and for providing emotional support to family members.

Transcribing Medical Prescriptions

- Nurses may need to receive new prescriptions for client care or medications by verbal or telephone order.

- When transcribing a prescription into a paper or electronic chart, nurses must:

  - Be sure to include all necessary elements of a prescription (date and time prescription was written; new client care prescription or medication including dosage, frequency, route of administration; and signature of nurse transcribing the prescription as well as the provider who verbally gave the prescription).

  - Follow institutional policy with regard to the time frame within which the provider must sign the order (usually within 24 hr).

  - Use strategies to prevent errors when taking a medical prescription that is given verbally or over the phone by the provider.

    - Repeat back the prescription given, making sure to include the medication name (spell if necessary), dosage, time, and route.

    - Question any prescription that may seem contraindicated due to a previous or concurrent prescription or client condition.

DISRUPTIVE BEHAVIOR

Overview

- Nurses experience incivility, lateral violence, and bullying at an alarming rate. The perpetrator may be a provider or a nursing colleague. Consequences of disruptive behavior include poor communication, which can negatively affect client safety and productivity, resulting in absenteeism, decreased job satisfaction, and staff turnover. Some nurses may choose to leave the profession due to these counterproductive behaviors.

- If disruptive behavior is allowed to continue, it is likely to escalate. Over time, it can be viewed as acceptable in that unit or department's culture.

- Types of Disruptive Behavior

  - Incivility is defined as an action that is rude, intimidating, and insulting. It includes teasing, joking, dirty looks, and uninvited touching.

  - Lateral violence is also known as horizontal abuse or horizontal hostility. It occurs between individuals who are at the same level within the organization. For example, a more experienced staff nurse may be abusive to a newly licensed nurse. Common behaviors include verbal abuse, undermining activities, sabotage, gossip, withholding information, and ostracism.

  - Bullying behavior is persistent and relentless and is aimed at an individual who has limited ability to defend himself or herself. Bullying occurs when the perpetrator is at a higher level than the victim, for example, a nurse manager to a staff nurse. It is abuse of power that makes the recipient feel threatened, disgraced, and vulnerable. For example, a nurse manger may demonstrate favoritism for another nurse by making unfair assignments or refusing a promotion.

  - Cyberbullying is a type of disruptive behavior using the Internet or other electronic means.

- Interventions to Deter Disruptive Behaviors
  - Create an environment of mutual respect among staff.
  - Model appropriate behavior.
  - Increase staff awareness about disruptive behavior.
  - Make staff aware that offensive online remarks about employers and coworkers is a form of bullying and is prohibited even if the nurse is off-duty and it is posted off-site from the facility.
  - Avoid making excuses for disruptive behavior.
  - Support zero tolerance for disruptive behavior.
  - Establish mechanisms for open communication between staff nurses and nurse managers.
  - Adopt policies that limit the risk of retaliation when disruptive behavior is reported.

ETHICAL PRACTICE

Overview

- Ethics has several definitions, but the foundation of ethics is based on an expected behavior of a certain group in relation to what is considered right and wrong.
- Morals are the values and beliefs held by a person that guide behavior and decision-making.
- Ethical theory analyzes varying philosophies, systems, ideas, and principles used to make judgments about what is right and wrong, good and bad. Two common types of ethical theory are utilitarianism and deontology.
- Ethical principles are standards of what is right or wrong with regard to important social values and norms. Ethical principles pertaining to the treatment of clients include:
  - Autonomy – the ability of the client to make personal decisions, even when those decisions may not be in the client's own best interest
  - Beneficence – the care that is in the best interest of the client
  - Fidelity – keeping one's promise to the client about care that was offered
  - Justice – fair treatment in matters related to physical and psychosocial care and use of resources
  - Nonmaleficence – the nurse's obligation to avoid causing harm to the client
  - Veracity – the nurse's duty to tell the truth
- Unusual or complex ethical issues may need to be dealt with by a facility's ethics committee.

Ethical Decision-Making in Nursing

- Ethical dilemmas are problems for which more than one choice can be made, and the choice is influenced by the values and beliefs of the decision-makers. These are common in health care, and nurses must be prepared to apply ethical theory and decision making.
- A problem is an ethical dilemma if:
  - It cannot be solved solely by a review of scientific data.
  - It involves a conflict between two moral imperatives.
  - The answer will have profound effect on the situation/client.

- Nurses have a responsibility to be advocates, and to identify and report ethical situations.
  - Doing so through the chain of command offers some protection against retribution.
  - Some state nurse associations offer protection for nurses who report substandard or unethical practice.
- Ethical decision-making is the process by which a decision is made about an ethical issue. Frequently, this requires a balance between science and morality. There are several steps in ethical decision-making:
  - Identify whether the issue is an ethical dilemma.
  - State the ethical dilemma, including all surrounding issues and individuals involved.
  - List and analyze all possible options for resolving the dilemma, and review implications of each option.
  - Select the option that is in concert with the ethical principle applicable to this situation, the decision maker's values and beliefs, and the profession's values set forth for client care. Justify why that one option was selected.
  - Apply this decision to the dilemma and evaluate the outcomes.
- The *American Nurses Association Code of Ethics for Nurses* (2001) and the *International Council of Nurses' Code of Ethics for Nurses* (2006) are commonly used by professional nurses. The *Code of Ethics for Licensed Practical/Vocational Nurses* issued by the National Association for Practical Nurse Education and Services also serves as a set of standards for Nursing Practice. Codes of ethics are available at the organizations' Web sites.
- The Uniform Determination of Death Act (UDDA) can be used to assist with end-of-life and organ donor issues.
  - The UDDA provides two formal definitions of death that were developed by the National Conference of Commissioners on Uniform State Laws. Death is determined by one of two criteria:
    - An irreversible cessation of circulatory and respiratory functions
    - Irreversible cessation of all functions of the entire brain, including the brain stem
  - A determination of death must be made in accordance with accepted medical standards.

THE NURSE'S ROLE IN ETHICAL DECISION-MAKING	
Nurse's Role	Examples
› An agent for the client facing an ethical decision	› Caring for an adolescent client who has to decide whether to undergo an abortion even though her parents believe it is wrong
	› Discussing options with parents who have to decide whether to consent to a blood transfusion for a child when their religion prohibits such treatment
› A decision-maker in regard to nursing practice	› Assigning staff nurses a higher client load than recommended because administration has cut the number of nurses per shift
	› Witnessing a surgeon discuss only surgical options with a client without informing the client about more conservative measures available

APPLICATION EXERCISES

1. A nurse manger is observing the actions of a nurse she is supervising. Which of the following actions by the nurse requires the nurse manager to intervene? (Select all that apply.)

_____ A. Reviewing the health care record of a client assigned to another nurse

_____ B. Making a copy of a client's most current laboratory results for the provider during rounds

_____ C. Providing information about a client's condition to hospital clergy

_____ D. Discussing a client's condition over the phone with an individual who has provided the client's information code

_____ E. Participating in walking rounds that involve the exchange of client-related information outside clients' rooms

2. A nurse is caring for a client who is being prepared for surgery. The client hands the nurse information about advance directives and states, "Here, I don't need this. I am too young to worry about life-sustaining measures and what I want done for me." Which of the following actions should the nurse take?

A. Return the papers to the admitting department with a note stating that the client does not wish to address the issue at this time.

B. Explain to the client that you never know what can happen during surgery and that he should fill the papers out "just in case."

C. Contact a client representative to talk with the client and offer additional information about the purpose of advance directives.

D. Inform the client that surgery cannot be conducted unless he completes the advance directives forms.

3. A nurse is serving as a preceptor to a newly licensed nurse and is explaining the role of the nurse as advocate. Which of the following situations illustrates the advocacy role? (Select all that apply.)

_____ A. Verifying that a client understands what is done during a cardiac catheterization

_____ B. Discussing treatment options for a terminal diagnosis

_____ C. Informing members of the health care team that a client has do-not-resuscitate status

_____ D. Reporting that a health team member on the previous shift did not provide care as prescribed

_____ E. Assisting a client to make a decision about his care based on the nurse's recommendations

4. A nurse manager is providing information to the nurses on the unit about ensuring client rights. Which of the following outlines the rights of individuals in health care settings?

    A. American Nurses Association Code of Ethics

    B. HIPAA

    C. Patient Self-Determination Act

    D. Patient Care Partnership

5. A nurse is reviewing a client's health care record and discovers that the client's do-not-resuscitate (DNR) order has expired. The client's condition is not stable. Which of the following actions should the nurse take?

    A. Assume that the client does not want to be resuscitated, and take no action if she experiences cardiac arrest.

    B. Write a note on the front of the provider order sheet asking that the DNR order be reordered.

    C. Anticipate that CPR will be instituted if the client goes into cardiopulmonary arrest.

    D. Call the provider to determine whether the order should be immediately reinstated.

6. A toddler is being treated in the emergency department following a head contusion from a fall. History reveals the toddler lives at home with only her mother. The provider's discharge instructions include waking the child up every hour during the night to assess for indications of a possible head injury. In which of the following situations should the nurse intervene and attempt to prevent discharge?

    A. The mother states she does not have insurance or money for a follow-up visit.

    B. The child states her head hurts and she wants to go home.

    C. The nurse smells alcohol on the mother's breath.

    D. The mother verbalizes fear about taking the child home and requests she be kept overnight.

7. A newly licensed nurse is preparing to insert an IV catheter in a client. Which of the following sources should the nurse use to review the procedure and the standard at which it should be performed?

    A. Web site

    B. Institutional policy and procedure manual

    C. More experienced nurse

    D. State nurse practice act

8. A nurse witnesses an assistive personnel (AP) under her supervision reprimanding a client for not using the urinal properly. The AP threatens to put a diaper on the client if he does not use the urinal more carefully next time. Which of the following torts is the AP committing?

A. Assault

B. Battery

C. False imprisonment

D. Invasion of privacy

9. A nurse is preparing to serve on a committee that will review the policy on disruptive behavior. Use the ATI Active Learning Template: Basic Concept to complete this item to include the following:

A. Related Content: Describe another term used for lateral violence.

B. Nursing Interventions: Describe at least four interventions to deter disruptive behavior.

APPLICATION EXERCISES KEY

1. A. **CORRECT:** To maintain confidentiality, client information is disseminated on a need-to-know basis only. A nurse who is not assigned to care for a client should not access the client's information.

    B. **CORRECT:** Paper copies of confidential information create a risk for breach of confidentiality.

    C. **CORRECT:** Information about a client's condition is disseminated on a need-to-know basis. It is inappropriate to share this information with the hospital clergy.

    D. INCORRECT: The nurse can share information with an individual who has been provided the information code.

    E. **CORRECT:** Sharing information in the hallway where it can be overheard by others can result in a breach of confidentiality.

    Ⓝ NCLEX® Connection: Management of Care, Assignment, Delegation and Supervision

2. A. INCORRECT: The nurse should advocate for the client by ensuring that the client understands the purpose of advance directives. Therefore, this action is inappropriate.

    B. INCORRECT: This response is nontherapeutic and can cause the client to be anxious about the surgery.

    C. **CORRECT:** The nurse should advocate for the client by ensuring that the client understands the purpose of advance directives. Seeking the assistance of a client representative to provide information to the client is an appropriate action.

    D. INCORRECT: This statement is untrue and is a barrier to therapeutic communication.

    Ⓝ NCLEX® Connection: Management of Care, Advance Directives

3. A. **CORRECT:** Ensuring that the client has given informed consent illustrates nurse advocacy.

    B. INCORRECT: Discussing treatment options is not within the scope of practice of the nurse.

    C. **CORRECT:** Ensuring that the client's care is consistent with his do-not-resuscitate status illustrates nurse advocacy.

    D. **CORRECT:** Ensuring that all clients receive proper care illustrates nurse advocacy.

    E. INCORRECT: Assisting a client to make decisions about his care based on nurse recommendations is inappropriate. The nurse should support the client in making his own decisions.

    Ⓝ NCLEX® Connection: Management of Care, Advocacy

4.   A. INCORRECT: The American Nurses Association Code of Ethics provides nurses with a set of standards for nursing practice.

   B. INCORRECT: The privacy rules of HIPAA ensure client privacy and confidentiality.

   C. INCORRECT: The Patient Self-Determination Act is federal legislation that requires that all clients admitted to a health care facility be asked whether they have advance directives.

   D. **CORRECT:** The Patient Care Partnership is a document that addresses clients' rights when receiving care.

   Ⓝ NCLEX® Connection: Management of Care, Client Rights

5.   A. INCORRECT: Without a current DNR order, the nurse must initiate emergency resuscitation, which most likely is not consistent with the client's wishes.

   B. INCORRECT: Without a current DNR order, the nurse must initiate emergency resuscitation, which most likely is not consistent with the client's wishes. Writing a note on the order sheet likely will result in a delay in resolving the problem.

   C. INCORRECT: Without a current DNR order, the nurse must initiate emergency resuscitation, which most likely is not consistent with the client's wishes.

   D. **CORRECT:** The nurse should immediately call the provider to determine whether the order should be reinstated. This is the action to take to be sure that the client's wishes are carried out.

   Ⓝ NCLEX® Connection: Management of Care, Advocacy

6.   A. INCORRECT: Lack of insurance does not warrant a delay in discharge, but it may indicate the need for referral for social services to assist with client needs.

   B. INCORRECT: The toddler's report of pain is an expected finding.

   C. **CORRECT:** It would be unsafe to discharge a toddler who requires hourly monitoring with a mother who may be chemically impaired.

   D. INCORRECT: Fear verbalized by the mother does not warrant denial in discharge. The nurse should allay the mother's fears by educating her about how to monitor the child and provide phone numbers for the mother to use.

   Ⓝ NCLEX® Connection: Management of Care, Advocacy

7. A. INCORRECT: A Web site may not provide information that is consistent with institutional policy.

   B. **CORRECT:** The institutional policy and procedure manual will provide instructions on how to perform the procedure that is consistent with established standards. Therefore, this is the resource the nurse should use.

   C. INCORRECT: A more experienced nurse on the unit may not perform the procedure according to the policy and procedure manual.

   D. INCORRECT: The nurse practice act identifies scope of practice and other aspects of the law, but it does not set standards for performance of a procedure.

   Ⓝ NCLEX® Connection: Management of Care, Information Technology

8. A. **CORRECT:** Assault is conduct that makes a person fear he or she will be harmed.

   B. INCORRECT: Battery is physical contact without a person's consent.

   C. INCORRECT: False imprisonment is restraining a person against his or her will. It includes the use of physical or chemical restraints, and refusing to allow a client to leave a facility

   D. INCORRECT: Invasion of privacy is the unauthorized release of a client's private information.

   Ⓝ NCLEX® Connection: Management of Care, Ethical Practice

9. *Using ATI Active Learning Template: Basic Concept*

   A. Related Content
      • Lateral violence is also known as horizontal abuse or horizontal hostility.

   B. Nursing Interventions
      • Create an environment of mutual respect among staff.
      • Model appropriate behavior.
      • Increase staff awareness about disruptive behavior.
      • Make staff aware that offensive online remarks about employers and coworkers are a form of bullying and is prohibited even if the nurse is off-duty and it is posted off-site of the facility.
      • Avoid making excuses for disruptive behavior.
      • Support zero tolerance for disruptive behavior.
      • Establish mechanisms for open communication between staff nurses and nurse managers.
      • Adopt policies that limit the risk of retaliation when disruptive behavior is reported.

   Ⓝ NCLEX® Connection: Management of Care, Concepts of Management

CHAPTER 4   Maintaining a Safe Environment

TOPICS

> QSEN Competencies in Nursing Programs
> Handling Infectious and Hazardous Materials
> Safe Use of Equipment
> Accident and Injury Prevention
> Home Safety
> Ergonomic Principles

NCLEX® CONNECTIONS

When reviewing the chapters in this unit, keep in mind the relevant sections of the NCLEX® outline, in particular:

Client Needs: Safety and Infection Control

> Relevant topics/tasks include:

» Accident/Injury Prevention

> Make an appropriate room assignment for the cognitively impaired client.

» Error Prevention

> Verify appropriateness and/or accuracy of a treatment order.

» Handling Hazardous and Infectious Materials

> Follow procedures for handling biohazardous materials.

» Home Safety

> Evaluate client care environment for fire/environmental hazards.

» Safe Use of Equipment

> Facilitate appropriate and safe use of equipment.

CHAPTER 4 Maintaining a Safe Environment

Overview

- Maintaining a safe environment refers to the precautions and considerations required to ensure that physical environments are safe for clients and staff.

- Knowing how to maintain client safety has been identified by the Institute of Medicine as a competency that graduates of nursing programs must possess.

- Quality and Safety Education for Nurses (QSEN) faculty propose that nursing education focus not only on the knowledge needed to provide safe care but also on the skills and attitudes that accompany this competency.

- To maintain a safe environment, nurses must have knowledge, skills, and attitude about:

  ○ QSEN Competencies

  ○ Handling infectious and hazardous materials

  ○ Safe use of equipment

  ○ Accident and injury prevention

  ○ Home safety

  ○ Ergonomic principles

QSEN COMPETENCIES IN NURSING PROGRAMS

- Concern about the quality and safety of health care in the United States has prompted numerous reports and initiatives designed to address this issue. Data from the Joint Commission identify poor communication as a key factor in the majority of sentinel events. The Institute of Medicine (IOM) report *To Err is Human: Building a Safer Health System* issued in 1999 spoke to the frequency of unnecessary deaths and preventable medical errors, and identified system failure as a major factor. Subsequent publications pointed to the need to redesign the provision of client care and to improve the education of students in health care programs.

  ○ The QSEN project identified specific competencies to include in each prelicensure nursing curriculum. These six competencies are now integral components of the curriculum of many nursing programs in the United States.

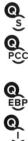

    ▪ Safety – The minimization of risk factors that could cause injury or harm while promoting quality care and maintaining a secure environment for clients, self, and others.

    ▪ Patient-Centered Care – The provision of caring and compassionate, culturally sensitive care that addresses clients' physiological, psychological, sociological, spiritual, and cultural needs, preferences, and values.

    ▪ Evidence-Based Practice – The use of current knowledge from research and other credible sources on which to base clinical judgment and client care.

    ▪ Informatics – The use of information technology as a communication and information-gathering tool that supports clinical decision-making and scientifically based nursing practice.

- Quality Improvement – Care-related and organizational processes that involve the development and implementation of a plan to improve health care services and better meet clients' needs.

- Teamwork and Collaboration – The delivery of client care in partnership with multidisciplinary members of the health care team to achieve continuity of care and positive client outcomes.

HANDLING INFECTIOUS AND HAZARDOUS MATERIALS

Overview

- Handling infectious and hazardous materials refers both to infection control procedures and to precautions for handling toxic, radioactive, or other hazardous materials.

- These safety measures are taken to protect the client, nurse, and other personnel and individuals from harmful materials and organisms.

- There are four levels of precautions (standard, airborne, droplet, contact) recommended for individuals coming in contact with clients carrying infectious organisms. Precautions consistent with the infectious organism should be followed as indicated.

- A manual containing material safety data sheets (MSDS) should be available in every workplace and should provide safety information, such as level of toxicity, handling and storage guidelines, and first aid and containment measures to take in case of accidental release of toxic, radioactive, or other dangerous materials. This manual should be available to all employees and may be housed in a location such as the emergency department of a hospital.

Infection Control

- Infection control is extremely important to prevent cross-contamination of communicable organisms and health care-associated infections.

  ○ Staff education on infection prevention and control is a responsibility of the nurse.

  ○ Facility policies and procedures should serve as a resource for proper implementation of infection prevention and control.

  ○ Clients suspected of, or diagnosed with, a communicable disease should be placed in the appropriate form of isolation.

  ○ The nurse should ensure that appropriate equipment is available and that isolation procedures are properly carried out by all health care team members.

  ○ Use of standard precautions by all members of the health care team should be enforced. Employees who are allergic to latex should have nonlatex gloves made available to them. A latex-free environment is provided for clients who have a latex allergy. Many health care facilities avoid the use of latex products unless there is no other alternative.

  ○ Hand hygiene facilities, as well as hand sanitizer, must be readily accessible to employees in client care areas.

○ Sturdy, moisture-resistant bags (usually red in color) should be used for soiled items, and the bags should be tied securely with a knot at the top. Double bagging is not cost effective and is unnecessary unless the outside of a bag becomes contaminated.

○ Retractable needles or needles with capping mechanisms, needleless syringes, and IV tubing with needleless connections should be available for use to prevent accidental needlesticks. Education on how to safely use these devices for administration of intermittent infusions will prevent misuse during client care and staff injuries from improper manipulation.

○ Sharps containers should be readily available in client care areas, and any needlestick involving an employee should be reported in accordance with facility policy and state law. An incident or occurrence report should also be filed. Most policies include testing of the client and nurse for blood-borne illnesses such as hepatitis and human immunodeficiency virus (HIV).

Hazardous Materials

- Nurses and other members of the health care team are at risk for exposure to hazardous materials.

- Employees have the right to refuse to work in hazardous working conditions if there is a clear threat to their health.

- Health care team members should follow occupational safety and health guidelines as set by the Occupational Safety and Health Administration (OSHA). Guidelines include

  ○ Providing each employee a work environment that is free from recognized hazards that can cause or are likely to cause death or serious physical harm

  ○ Making protective gear accessible to employees working under hazardous conditions or with hazardous materials (antineoplastic medications, sterilization chemicals)

  ○ Providing measurement devices and keeping records that document an employee's level of exposure over time to hazardous materials, such as radiation from x-rays

  ○ Providing education and recertification opportunities to each employee regarding these rules and regulations, such as handling of hazardous materials

  ○ Maintaining material safety data sheets (MSDSs) and ensuring their availability to all employees

  ○ Designating an institutional hazardous materials (HAZMAT) response team that responds to hazardous events

Handling Infectious and Hazardous Materials

- Members of the health care team must clean and maintain equipment that is shared by several clients on a unit (blood pressure cuffs, thermometers, pulse oximeters).

- Keep designated equipment in the rooms of clients who are on contact precautions.

- Use standard precautions at all times.

- Employ proper hand hygiene techniques.

- Use needlestick precautions when handling needles and sharps.

- Maintain knowledge of rules and regulations and proper procedures for handling infectious/hazardous materials (use of red biohazard bag for disposal of contaminated materials, proper use of puncture-proof containers for sharps).

SAFE USE OF EQUIPMENT

Overview

- Safe use of equipment refers to appropriate operation of health care-related equipment by trained staff. Equipment-related injuries may occur as a result of malfunction, disrepair, or mishandling of mechanical equipment.

- Nurses must ensure that they have the competence necessary to use equipment for tasks that fall within their scope of practice. Nurses should use equipment only after receiving sufficient instruction.

- Equipment should be regularly inspected by the engineering or maintenance department and by the user prior to use. Faulty equipment (frayed cords, disrepair) can start a fire or cause an electrical shock and should be removed from use and reported immediately per the health care agency's policy.

Safe Use of Equipment

- Nurses' responsibilities related to equipment safety include

    - Learning how to use and maintaining competency in the use of equipment

    - Checking that equipment is accurately set and functioning properly (oxygen, nasogastric suction) at the beginning and during each shift

    - Ensuring that electrical equipment is grounded (three-pronged plug and grounded outlet) to decrease the risk for electrical shock

    - Ensuring that outlet covers are used in environments with individuals at risk for sticking items into them

    - Unplugging equipment using the plug, not the cord, to prevent bending the plug prongs, which increases the risk for electrical shock

    - Ensuring that life-support equipment is plugged into outlets designated to be powered by a backup generator during power outages

    - Disconnecting all electrical equipment prior to cleaning

    - Ensuring that all pumps (general and PCA) have free-flow protection to prevent an overdose of fluids or medications

    - Ensuring that outlets are not overcrowded and that extension cords are used only when absolutely necessary (if they must be used in an open area, tape the cords to the floor)

    - Using all equipment only as it is intended

    - Immediately removing nonworking equipment from the client care area and sending it to the proper department for repair or disposal

ACCIDENT AND INJURY PREVENTION

Overview

- Preventing injury is a major nursing responsibility. Many factors affect a client's ability to protect himself. Those factors include the client's:
  - ○ Age (the young and the old are at greater risk)
  - ○ Mobility
  - ○ Cognitive and sensory awareness
  - ○ Emotional state
  - ○ Lifestyle and safety awareness
- All health care workers must be aware of:
  - ○ How to assess for and recognize clients at risk for safety issues
  - ○ Procedural safety guidelines
  - ○ Protocols for responding to dangerous situations
  - ○ Security plans
  - ○ Identification and documentation of incidents and responses per health care agency policy

Falls

- Prevention of client falls is a major nursing priority. All clients admitted to health care institutions should be assessed for risk factors related to falls, and based on the assessment, preventative measures should be implemented.

- Older adult clients may be at an increased risk for falls due to decreased strength, impaired mobility and balance, and endurance limitations combined with decreased sensory perception.
- Other clients at increased risk include those who have decreased visual acuity, generalized weakness, urinary frequency, gait and balance problems (cerebral palsy, injury, multiple sclerosis), and cognitive dysfunction. Adverse effects of medications (orthostatic hypotension, drowsiness) also can increase the risk for falls.

- Clients are at greater risk for falls when multiple risk factors are present.
- Prevention of Falls
  - ○ Complete a fall risk assessment on the client upon admission and at regular intervals.
  - ○ The plan for each client is individualized based on the fall risk assessment.
  - ○ For example, if the client has orthostatic hypotension, instruct the client to avoid getting up too quickly, to sit on the side of the bed for a few seconds prior to standing, and to stand at the side of the bed for a few seconds prior to walking.
  - ○ General measures to prevent falls include the following:
    - ▪ Be sure the client knows how to use the call light, that it is in reach, and encourage its use.
    - ▪ Respond to call lights in a timely manner.

- Orient the client to the setting (grab bars, call light), and ensure that the client understands how to use all assistive devices and can locate necessary items.

- Place clients at risk for falls near the nursing station.

- Ensure that bedside tables and overbed tables and frequently used items (telephone, water, tissues, call light) are within the client's reach.

- Maintain the bed in low position.

- Keep bed rails up and the bed in the low position for clients who are sedated, unconscious, or otherwise compromised.

- Avoid using full side bed rails for clients who get out of bed or attempt to get out of bed without assistance.

- Provide the client with nonskid footwear.

- Keep the floor free from clutter with a clear path to the bathroom (no scatter rugs, cords, furniture).

- Keep assistive devices (glasses, walkers, transfer devices) nearby after validation of safe use by the client and family.

- Educate the client and family/caregivers on identified risks and the plan of care.

- Lock wheels on beds, wheelchairs, and carts to prevent the device from rolling during transfers or stops.

- Use chair or bed sensors to alert staff of independent ambulation for clients at risk for getting up unattended.

- Report and document all incidents per the health care agency's policy. This provides valuable information that may be helpful in preventing similar incidents.

- To evaluate incidence of client falls, a formula based on 1,000 client days can be used. The formula is the number of client falls ÷ number of client days x 1,000 = fall rate per 1,000 client days. Using this formula, a facility can compare its fall rates to other facilities.

Seizures

- A seizure is a sudden surge of electrical activity in the brain. Seizures may occur at any time during a person's life and may be due to epilepsy, fever, or a variety of medical conditions. Partial seizures are due to electrical surges in one part of the brain, and generalized seizures involve the entire brain.

Seizure Precautions

- Seizure precautions (measures to protect the client from injury should a seizure occur) are taken for clients who have a history of seizures that involve the entire body and/or result in unconsciousness.

  ○ Ensure that rescue equipment, including oxygen, an oral airway, and suction equipment, is at the bedside. A saline lock may be placed for intravenous access if the client is at high risk for experiencing a generalized seizure.

  ○ Inspect the client's environment for items that may cause injury in the event of a seizure, and remove items that are not necessary for current treatment.

  ○ Assist the client who is at risk for a seizure with ambulation and transfers to reduce the risk of injury.

○ Advise all caregivers and family not to put anything in the client's mouth in the event of a seizure (except in status epilepticus, where an airway is needed).

○ Advise all caregivers and family not to restrain the client in the event of a seizure. Instead, ensure the client's safety by lowering him to the floor or bed, protecting his head, removing nearby furniture, providing privacy, putting the client on his side with his head slightly flexed forward if possible, and loosening clothing to prevent injury and promote dignity.

○ In the event of a seizure, stay with the client, protect the client from injury, and call for help.

○ Note the duration of the seizure and the sequence and type of movement.

○ After a seizure, explain what happened to the client, and provide comfort, understanding, and a quiet environment for recovery.

○ Document the seizure in the client's record along with any precipitating behaviors and a description of the event (movements, any injuries, length of seizure, aura, postictal state), and report it to the provider.

Seclusion and Restraints

• Seclusion and restraints are used to prevent clients from injuring themselves or others.

○ Seclusion is the placement of a client in a room that is private, isolated, and safe. Seclusion is used for clients who are at risk for injuring themselves or others.

○ Physical restraint involves the application of a device that limits the client's movement. A restraint may limit the movement of the entire body or a body part.

○ Chemical restraints are medications used to control the client's disruptive behavior.

• Risks Associated with Use of Restraints

○ Deaths by asphyxiation and strangulation have occurred with restraints.

○ The client may also experience complications related to immobility, such as pressure ulcers, urinary and fecal incontinence, and pneumonia.

• Legal Considerations

○ Nurses should understand agency polices as well as federal and state laws that govern the use of restraints and seclusion.

○ False imprisonment means the confinement of person without his consent. Improper use of restraints may subject the nurse to charges of false imprisonment.

• Guidelines

○ In general, seclusion and/or restraints should be ordered for the shortest duration necessary and only if less restrictive measures have proved insufficient. They are for the physical protection of the client, or the protection of other clients or staff.

○ A client may voluntarily request temporary seclusion in cases where the environment is disturbing or seems too stimulating.

○ The use of restraints is a difficult adjustment for both the client and the family. The client loses his freedom and may be embarrassed and experience low self-esteem and depression. The nurse can allay some of the concerns by explaining the purpose of the restraint and that the restraint is only temporary.

- Seclusion and/or restraints must never be used for
  - Convenience of the staff
  - Punishment for the client
  - Clients who are extremely physically or mentally unstable
  - Clients who cannot tolerate the decreased stimulation of a seclusion room
- PRN prescriptions for restraints are not permitted.
- Restraints should
  - Never interfere with treatment
  - Restrict movement as little as is necessary to ensure safety
  - Fit properly
  - Be easily changed to decrease the chance of injury and to provide for the greatest level of dignity
- When all other less restrictive means have been tried to prevent a client from harming self or others, the following must occur for seclusion or restraints to be used:
  - The treatment must be prescribed by the provider based on a face-to-face assessment of the client.
    - In an emergency situation in which there is immediate risk to the client or others, the nurse may place a client in restraints. The nurse must obtain a prescription from the provider as soon as possible in accordance with agency policy (usually within 1 hr).
  - The prescription must specify the reason for the restraint, the type of restraint, the location of the restraint, how long the restraint may be used, and the type of behaviors demonstrated by the client that warrant use of the restraint.
  - The provider must rewrite the prescription, specifying the type of restraint, every 24 hr or the frequency of time specified by facility policy.
- Nursing Responsibilities
  - Obtain a prescription from the provider for the restraint. If the client is at risk for harming self or others and a restraint is applied prior to consulting the provider, ensure that notification of the provider occurs in accordance with facility protocol.
  - Conduct neurosensory checks every 2 hours to include
    - Circulation
    - Sensation
    - Mobility
  - Offer food and fluids.
  - Provide with means for hygiene and elimination.
  - Monitor vital signs.
  - Provide range of motion of extremities.
  - Follow agency polices regarding restraints, including the need for a signed consent from the client or guardian.
  - Review the manufacturer's instructions for correct application.
  - Remove or replace restraints frequently.
  - Pad bony prominences.

- Use a quick-release knot to tie the restraint to the bed frame.
- Ensure that the restraint is loose enough for range of motion and has enough room to fit two fingers between the device and the client.
- Regularly assess the need for continued use of the restraints.
- Never leave the client unattended without the restraint.
- Documentation
  - The behavior or precipitating events that make the restraint necessary
  - Attempts to use alternatives to restraints and the client's response
  - The client's level of consciousness
  - Type of restraint used and location
  - Education/explanations to the client and family
  - Exact time of application and removal
  - The client's behavior while restrained
  - Type and frequency of care (range of motion, neurosensory checks, removal, integumentary checks)
  - The client's response when the restraint is removed
  - Medication administration

Fire Safety

- Fires in health care facilities are usually due to problems related to electrical or anesthetic equipment. Unauthorized smoking may also be the case of a fire.
- All staff must be instructed in fire response procedures, which include knowing the following:
  - Location of exits, fire extinguishers, and oxygen turnoff valves
  - Evacuation plan for the unit and facility
- Fire response in health care settings always follows the RACE sequence:
  - R: Rescue – Rescue and protect clients in close proximity to the fire by evacuating them to a safer location. Ambulatory clients can walk unattended to a safe location.
  - A: Alarm – Activate the facility alarm system.
  - C: Contain – Contain the fire by closing doors and windows as well as turning off any sources of oxygen. Clients who are on life support are ventilated with a bag-valve mask.
  - E: Extinguish – Extinguish the fire if possible using an appropriate fire extinguisher.
    - There are three classes of fire extinguisher.
      - Class A is for paper, wood, upholstery, rags, or other types of trash fires.
      - Class B is for flammable liquids and gas fires.
      - Class C is for electrical fires.
    - To use a fire extinguisher, follow the PASS sequence:
      - P: Pull – Pull the pin.
      - A: Aim – Aim at the base of the fire.
      - S: Squeeze – Squeeze the levers.
      - S: Sweep – Sweep the extinguisher from side to side, covering the area of the fire.

HOME SAFETY

Overview

- In addition to taking measures to prevent injury to clients in a health care setting, nurses play a pivotal role in promoting safety in the client's home and community. Nurses often collaborate with the client, family, and members of the interprofessional team (social workers, occupational therapists, physical therapists) to promote the client's safety.

- A number of factors contribute to the client's risk for injury. These factors include the client's

  - Age and developmental status
  - Mobility and balance
  - Knowledge about safety hazards
  - Sensory and cognitive awareness
  - Communication skills
  - Home and work environment
  - Community

- To initiate a plan of care, the nurse must identify risk factors using a risk assessment tool and complete a nursing history, physical examination, and home hazard appraisal.

Safety Risks Based on Age and Developmental Status

- The age and developmental status of the client creates specific safety risks.

RISK	PREVENTION EDUCATION
Infants and toddlers	
› Aspiration	› Keep all small objects out of reach.
	› Check toys for loose parts.
	› Do not feed infants hard candy, peanuts, popcorn, or whole or sliced pieces of hot dog.
	› Do not place infants in the supine position while feeding or prop the bottle.
	› A pacifier (if used) should be constructed of one piece.
› Burns	› Test the temperature of formula and bath water.
	› Place pots on back burners and turn handles away from the front of stove.
	› Supervise use of faucets.
	› Keep matches and lighters out of reach.

RISK	PREVENTION EDUCATION
Infants and toddlers	
› Suffocation	› Keep plastic bags out of reach.
	› Teach the "back to sleep" mnemonic and always place infants on back to rest.
	› Make sure crib mattress fits snugly and that crib slats are no more than 2 ⅜ inches apart.
	› Never leave an infant or toddler alone in the bathtub.
	› Remove crib toys such as mobiles from over the bed as soon as the infant begins to push up.
	› Keep latex balloons away from infants and toddlers.
	› Fence swimming pools, and use a locked gate.
	› Begin swimming lessons when the child's developmental status allows for protective responses such as closing mouth under water.
	› Keep toilet lids down and bathroom doors closed.
› Poisoning	› Keep house plants and cleaning agents out of reach.
	› Place poisons, paint, and gasoline in locked cabinets.
	› Inspect and remove sources of lead, such as paint chips, and provide parents with information about prevention of lead poisoning.
	› Keep medications in child-proof containers and locked up.
	› Dispose of medications that are no longer used or are out of date.
› Falls	› Keep crib and playpen rails up.
	› Never leave infants unattended on a changing table or other high surface.
	› Restrain when in high chair, swing, stroller.
	› Place in a low bed when toddler starts to climb.
› Motor vehicle/ Injury	› Place infants and toddlers in a rear-facing car seat until 2 years of age or until they exceed the height and weight limit of the car seat. Then they can sit in a forward-facing seat.
	› A car seat with a five-point harness should be used for both infants and children.
	› All car seats should be federally approved and be placed in the back seat.
Preschoolers and school-age children	
› Drowning	› Be sure the child has learned to swim and knows the rules of water safety.
	› Place locked fences around home and neighborhood pools.
› Motor vehicle/ Injury	› Use booster seats for children who are less than 4 feet, 9 inches tall and weigh less than 40 lb (usually 4 to 8 years old). The child should be able to sit with his back against the car seat, and his legs should dangle over the seat. If car has passenger airbag, place children under 12 years in back seat.
	› Use seat belts properly after booster seats are no longer necessary.
	› Ensure the use of protective equipment for sports or bike riding.
	› Supervise and teach safe use of equipment.
	› Teach the child to play in safe areas.
	› Teach the child safety rules of the road.
	› Teach the child what to do if approached by stranger.
	› Begin sex education for school-age children.

RISK	PREVENTION EDUCATION
Preschoolers and school-age children	
› Burns	› Reduce setting on water heater to no higher than 120° F.
	› Teach dangers of playing with matches, fireworks, firearms.
	› Teach school-age children how to properly use microwave and other cooking instruments.
› Poison	› Teach the child about the hazards of alcohol, prescription and nonprescription medications, and illegal drugs.
	› Keep potentially dangerous substances out of reach.
Adolescents	
› Motor vehicle/ Injury	› Ensure the teen has completed a driver education course.
	› Set rules for the number of people allowed to ride in the car and for seat belt use
	› Tell the teen to call for a ride home if a driver is impaired.
	› Reinforce teaching on proper use of protective equipment when participating in sports.
	› Be alert to signs of depression.
	› Teach about the hazards of firearms and safety precautions with firearms.
	› Teach to check water depth before diving.
› Burns	› Teach to use sunblock and protective clothing.
	› Teach dangers of sunbathing and tanning beds.
	› Educate on the hazards of smoking.

- Safety Risks and Prevention Measures for Young and Middle Age Adults

  o Motor vehicle crashes are the most common cause of death and injury to the adult. Occupational injuries contribute to the injury and death rate of the adult. High consumption of alcohol and suicide are also major concerns for adults.

  o Nurses can promote client safety for young and middle age adults by

    ▪ Reminding clients to drive defensively and to not drive after drinking alcohol

    ▪ Reinforcing teaching about the long-term effects related to high alcohol consumption

    ▪ Being attuned to behaviors that suggest the presence of depression and/or thoughts of suicide, and referring clients as appropriate

    ▪ Encouraging clients to become proactive about safety in the workplace

    ▪ Ensuring that clients understand the hazards of excessive sun exposure and the need to protect the skin with the use of sun-blocking agents and protective clothing

 - Safety Risks and Prevention Measures for Older Adults

  o The rate at which age-related changes occur varies greatly among older adults.

  o Many older adults are able to maintain a lifestyle that promotes independence and the ability to protect themselves from safety hazards.

- ○ Risk factors for injuries for older adults
  - ▪ Physical, cognitive, and sensory changes
    - □ Changes in the musculoskeletal and neurological systems (falls)
    - □ Vision and/or hearing impairment (falls)
    - □ Frequent trips to the bathroom at night because of nocturia and incontinence (falls)
    - □ A decrease in tactile sensitivity (burns, other types of tissue injury)
- ○ When the client demonstrates factors that increase the risk for injury (regardless of age), a home hazard evaluation should be conducted by a nurse, a physical therapist, and/or occupational therapist. The client is made aware of the environmental factors that may pose a risk to safety and suggested modifications.
- ○ Modifications that can be made to improve home safety
  - ▪ Removing items that could cause the client to trip, such as throw rugs and loose carpets
  - ▪ Placing electrical cords and extension cords against a wall behind furniture
  - ▪ Making sure that steps and sidewalks are in good repair
  - ▪ Placing grab bars near the toilet and in the tub or shower, and installing a stool riser
  - ▪ Using a nonskid mat in the tub or shower
  - ▪ Placing a shower chair in the shower
  - ▪ Ensuring that lighting is adequate both inside and outside of the home

Home Safety Plan

- Home fires continue to be a major cause of death and injury for people of all ages. Nurses should educate clients about the importance of a home safety plan.
- The plan includes the following:
  - ○ Keep emergency numbers near the phone for prompt use in the event of an emergency of any type.
  - ○ Ensure that the number and placement of fire extinguishers and smoke alarms are adequate and that they are operable.
  - ○ Set a specific time to routinely change the batteries in the smoke alarms (in the fall when the clocks are set back to standard time and spring when reset at daylight saving time).
  - ○ Have a family exit and meeting plan for fires that is reviewed and practiced regularly.
  - ○ Be sure to close windows and doors if able.
  - ○ Exit a smoke-filled area by covering the mouth and nose with a damp cloth and getting down as close to the floor as possible.
  - ○ Review with clients of all ages that in the event that the client's clothing or skin is on fire "stop, drop, and roll" should be used to extinguish the fire.

- Safe Use of Oxygen in the Home

  - If oxygen is being used in the home, oxygen safety measures should be reviewed. Oxygen can cause materials to combust more easily and burn more rapidly, so the client and family must be provided with information on use of the oxygen delivery equipment and the dangers of combustion.

  - The teaching plan should include the following:

    - Use and store oxygen equipment according to the manufacturer's recommendations.

    - Place a "No Smoking" sign in a conspicuous place near the front door of the home. A sign may also be placed on the door to the client's bedroom.

    - Inform the client and family of the danger of smoking in the presence of oxygen. Family members and visitors who smoke should do so outside the home.

    - Ensure that electrical equipment is in good repair and well grounded.

    - Replace bedding that generates static electricity (wool, nylon, synthetics) with items made from cotton.

    - Keep flammable materials, such as heating oil and nail polish remover, away from the client when oxygen is in use.

    - Follow general measures for fire safety in the home, such as having a fire extinguisher readily available and an established exit route should a fire occur.

Additional Risks in the Home and Community

- Additional risks in the home and community include passive smoking, carbon monoxide poisoning, and food poisoning. Bioterrorism has also become a concern, making disaster plans a mandatory part of community safety.

- Nurses should teach clients about the dangers of these additional risks.

  - Passive Smoking

    - Passive smoking is the unintentional inhalation of tobacco smoke.

    - Exposure to nicotine and other toxins places people at risk for numerous diseases, including cancer, heart disease, and lung infections.

    - Low birth weight, prematurity, stillbirths, and sudden infant death syndrome (SIDS) have been associated with maternal smoking.

    - Passive smoking is associated with childhood development of bronchitis, pneumonia, and middle ear infections.

    - For children who have asthma, exposure to passive smoke can result in an increase in the frequency and the severity of asthma attacks.

    - Nurses should inform clients who smoke and their families about the following:

      - The hazards of smoking

      - Available resources to stop smoking (smoking-cessation programs, medication support, self-help groups)

      - The effect that visiting individuals who smoke or riding in the automobile of a smoker has on a nonsmoker

- ○ Carbon Monoxide

  - Carbon monoxide is a very dangerous gas because it binds with hemoglobin and ultimately reduces the oxygen supplied to tissues in the body.

  - Carbon monoxide cannot be seen, smelled, or tasted.

  - Indications of carbon monoxide poisoning include nausea, vomiting, headache, weakness, and unconsciousness.

  - Death may occur with prolonged exposure.

  - Measures to prevent carbon monoxide poisoning include ensuring proper ventilation when using fuel-burning devices (lawn mowers, wood-burning and gas fireplaces, charcoal grills).

  - Gas-burning furnaces, water heaters, and appliances should be inspected annually.

  - Flues and chimneys should be unobstructed.

  - Carbon monoxide detectors should be installed and inspected regularly.

- ○ Food Poisoning

  - Food poisoning is a major cause of illness in the United States.

  - Most food poisoning is caused by some type of bacteria, such as *Escherichia coli*, *Listeria monocytogenes*, and *Salmonella*.

  - Healthy individuals usually recover from the illness in a few days.

  - Very young, very old, pregnant women, and immunocompromised individuals are at risk for complications.

  - Clients who are especially at risk are instructed to follow a low-microbial diet.

  - Most food poisoning occurs because of unsanitary food practice.

  - Proper hand hygiene, ensuring that meat and fish are cooked to the correct temperature, handling raw and fresh food separately to avoid cross-contamination, and refrigerating perishable items are measures that may prevent food poisoning.

- ○ Bioterrorism

  - Bioterrorism is the dissemination of harmful toxins, bacteria, viruses, or pathogens for the purpose of causing illness or death.

  - Anthrax, variola, *Clostridium botulinum*, and *Yersinia pestis* are examples of types of agents used by terrorists.

  - Nurses and other health professionals must be prepared to respond to an attack by being proficient in early detection, recognizing the causative agent, identifying the affected community, and providing early treatment to affected people. For more information, go to the website of the Association of Professionals in Infection Control and Epidemiology (http://www.apic.org/).

ERGONOMIC PRINCIPLES

Overview

- Ergonomics are the factors or qualities in an object's design and/or use that contribute to comfort, safety, efficiency, and ease of use.
- Body mechanics is the proper use of muscles to maintain balance, posture, and body alignment when performing a physical task. Nurses use body mechanics when providing care to clients by lifting, bending, and carrying out the activities of daily living.
- The risk of injury to the client and the nurse is reduced with the use of good body mechanics. Whenever possible, mechanical lift devices should be used to lift and transfer clients. Many health care agencies have "no manual lift" and "no solo lift" policies.

Safety Measures

- Guidelines to Prevent Injury
  - Know your agency's policies regarding lifting.
  - Plan ahead for activities that require lifting, transfer, or ambulation of a client, and ask other staff members to be ready to assist at the time planned.
  - Be aware that the safest way to lift a client may be with the use of assistive equipment.
  - Rest between heavy lifting activities to decrease muscle fatigue.
  - Maintain good posture and exercise regularly to increase the strength of arm, leg, back, and abdominal muscles so these activities require less energy.
  - Use smooth movements when lifting and moving clients to prevent injury through sudden or jerky muscle movements.
  - When standing for long periods of time, flex the hip and knee through use of a foot rest. When sitting for long periods of time, keep the knees slightly higher than the hips.
  - Avoid repetitive movements of the hands, wrists, and shoulders. Take a break every 15 to 20 min to flex and stretch joints and muscles.
  - Maintain good posture (head and neck in straight line with pelvis) to avoid neck flexion and hunched shoulders, which can cause impingement of nerves in the neck.
  - Avoid twisting the spine or bending at the waist (flexion) to minimize the risk for injury.
- Center of Gravity
  - The center of gravity is the center of a mass.
  - Weight is a quantity of matter acted on by the force of gravity.
  - To lift an object, the nurse must overcome the weight of the object and know the center of gravity of the object.
  - When the human body is in the upright position, the center of gravity is the pelvis.
  - When an individual moves, the center of gravity shifts.
  - The closer the line of gravity is to the center of the base of support, the more stable the individual is.
  - To lower the center of gravity, bend the hips and knees.

- Lifting
  - Use the major muscle groups to prevent back strain, and tighten the abdominal muscles to increase support to the back muscles.
  - Distribute the weight between the large muscles of the arms and legs to decrease the strain on any one muscle group and avoid strain on smaller muscles.
  - When lifting an object from the floor, flex the hips, knees, and back. Get the object to thigh level keeping the knees bent and straightening the back. Stand up while holding the object as close as possible to the body, bringing the load to the center of gravity to increase stability and decrease back strain.
  - Use assistive devices whenever possible, and seek assistance whenever it is needed.
- Pushing or Pulling a Load
  - Widen the base of support.
  - When opportunity allows, pull objects toward the center of gravity rather than pushing away.
  - If pushing, move the front foot forward, and if pulling, move the rear leg back to promote stability.
  - Face the direction of movement when moving a client.
  - Use own body as a counterweight when pushing or pulling, which makes the movement easier.
  - Sliding, rolling, and pushing require less energy than lifting and have less risk for injury.
  - Avoid twisting the thoracic spine and bending the back while the hips and knees are straight.
- Transfers and Use of Assistive Devices
  - Assess the client's ability to help with transfers (balance, muscle strength, endurance).
  - Determine the need for additional personnel or assistive devices (transfer belt, hydraulic lift, sliding board).
  - Assess and monitor the client's use of mobility aids (canes, walkers, crutches).
  - Include assistance or mobility aids needed for safe transfers and ambulation in plan of care.

APPLICATION EXERCISES

1. A home health nurse is assessing the safety of a client's home. Which of the following factors may increase the client's risk for falls? (Select all that apply.)

_____   A. History of a previous fall

_____   B. Reduced vision

_____   C. Impaired memory

_____   D. Takes rosuvastatin (Crestor)

_____   E. Wears house slippers

_____   F. Kyphosis

2. A client is brought back to the unit after a total hip arthroplasty. The client is confused, is moving his leg into positions that could dislocate the new hip joint, and he repeatedly attempts to get out of bed. Which of the following actions should the nurse take? (Select all that apply.)

_____   A. Apply arm and leg restraints immediately.

_____   B. Get an order from the provider.

_____   C. Have a family member sign the consent for restraints.

_____   D. Use a square knot to secure the restraints to the bed frame.

_____   E. Ensure that only one finger can be inserted between the restraint and the client.

3. A nurse is observing a newly licensed nurse and an assistive personnel (AP) pull a client up in bed using a drawsheet. Which of the following actions by the newly licensed nurse indicates a need for further education?

A. The nurse spreads his legs apart.

B. The nurse uses his body weight to counter the client's weight.

C. The nurse's feet are facing inward, toward the center of the bed.

D. The nurse uses the muscles in his arms to lift the client off the bed using the drawsheet.

4. An assistive personnel (AP) reports that a client's finger-stick blood glucose reading 30 min before lunch is 58 mg/dL. The client's morning finger-stick blood glucose was 285 mg/dL. The client is asymptomatic for hypoglycemia, and his next dose of insulin is scheduled to be administered at this time. Which of the following actions should the nurse take first?

    A. Recalibrate the glucometer, and recheck the client's blood glucose.

    B. Have the laboratory draw a stat serum glucose.

    C. Inform the AP to give the client 120 mL of orange juice.

    D. Administer insulin as prescribed.

5. A staff nurse is reviewing the hospital's fire safety policies and procedures with newly hired assistive personnel. The nurse is describing what to do when there is a fire in a client's trash can. Which of the following statements should the nurse include? (Select all that apply.)

    _____ A. The first step is to pull the alarm.

    _____ B. Use a Class C fire extinguisher to put out the fire.

    _____ C. Instruct ambulatory clients to evacuate to a safe place.

    _____ D Pull the pin on the fire extinguisher prior to use.

    _____ E. Close all doors.

6. A nurse manager is preparing to discuss electrical safety with the nurses on her unit. List the information that should be included in the discussion for each of the following aspects of safety. Use the ATI Active Learning Template: Basic Concept to complete this item. In the section Underlying Principles, identify the frequency in which the nurse should check equipment, and list four measures to prevent electrical shock.

APPLICATION EXERCISES KEY

1. A. **CORRECT:** A client who has had a previous fall is at risk for another fall.

    B. **CORRECT:** Reduced vision makes it difficult for the client to avoid mishaps with equipment and furniture.

    C. **CORRECT:** A client who has impaired memory may not ask for help with ambulation or ADLs.

    D. INCORRECT: This medication does not place the client at risk for falls.

    E. **CORRECT:** House slippers may not provide adequate traction and support for safe ambulation.

    F. **CORRECT:** Kyphosis, which is a type of curvature of the spine, alters a client posture and center of balance and may place the client at risk for falls.

    Ⓝ NCLEX® Connection: Safety and Infection Control, Home Safety

2. A. **CORRECT:** If a client is in imminent danger of harming himself, the nurse can apply restraints immediately.

    B. **CORRECT:** The nurses must obtain an order from the provider as soon as possible, typically within 1 hr.

    C. **CORRECT:** A family member must sign a consent for the restraint.

    D. INCORRECT: A quick-release knot must be used to secure the restraint to the bed frame.

    E. INCORRECT: The distance between the restraint and the client should be two finger widths.

    Ⓝ NCLEX® Connection: Safety and Infection Control, Use of Restraints/Safety Devices

3. A. INCORRECT: When the nurse pulls a client up in bed, he should spread his legs apart to create a wide base of support.

    B. INCORRECT: The nurse should use his body weight to counter the client's weight to make pulling easier.

    C. **CORRECT:** This action by the nurse requires intervention. The nurse's feet should be pointing at the head of the bed instead of the center of the bed.

    D. INCORRECT: The nurse should use the larger muscles of the arm to lift the client.

    Ⓝ NCLEX® Connection: Management of Care, Assignment, Delegation and Supervision

NURSING LEADERSHIP AND MANAGEMENT

4. A. **CORRECT:** Because the blood glucose was 285 mg/dL a few hours ago, it is unlikely that the blood glucose is 58 mg/dL at this time. Therefore, the nurse should recalibrate the glucometer and recheck the client's blood glucose.

    B. INCORRECT: This is not the first action the nurse should take. It may be unnecessary to take this action and may add cost to client care.

    C. INCORRECT: This is not the first action the nurse should take. Because the client's blood glucose was high a few hours ago, it is unlikely that the blood glucose is low enough to warrant giving the client orange juice. If the client's blood glucose is very low, the nurse may take this action.

    D. INCORRECT: This is not the first action the nurse should take. The nurse should have an accurate blood glucose reading prior to administering insulin.

    Ⓝ NCLEX® Connection: Safety and Infection Control, Safe Use of Equipment

5. A. INCORRECT: When a fire occurs in a client's room, the first step for the employee to take is to remove or evacuate the client from the room. The employee should know the RACE sequence: rescue the client, pull the alarm, contain the fire, and then extinguish the fire.

    B. INCORRECT: Class A fire extinguishers are used for paper, wood, and cloth.

    C. **CORRECT:** Ambulatory clients can walk by themselves to a safe place.

    D. **CORRECT:** The fire extinguisher PASS sequence is pull the pin, aim at the base of the fire, squeeze the lever, and sweep the fire extinguisher from side to side.

    E. **CORRECT:** The employee should close all doors to contain the fire.

    Ⓝ NCLEX® Connection: Safety and Infection Control, Accident/Error/Injury Prevention

6. *Using ATI Active Learning Template: Basic Concept*
    - Underlying Principles
      - The nurse should check all equipment at the beginning and end of each shift.
      - Measures to Prevent Electrical Shock
        - Ensure that all electrical equipment has a three-way plug and grounded outlet.
        - Ensure that outlet covers are used in areas such as pediatric and mental health units.
        - When unplugging equipment, grasp the plug, not the cord.
        - Disconnect all equipment prior to cleaning.
        - Ensure that outlets are not overcrowded.
        - Use extension cords only when absolute necessary; if used in an open area, tape the cords to the floor.

    Ⓝ NCLEX® Connection: Safety and Infection Control, Accident/Error/Injury Prevention

CHAPTER 5   Facility Protocols

TOPICS

› Reporting Incidents
› Disaster Planning and Emergency Response
› Security Plans

NCLEX® CONNECTIONS

When reviewing the chapters in this unit, keep in mind the relevant sections of the NCLEX® outline, in particular:

Client Needs: Safety and Infection Control

› Relevant topics/tasks include:

  » Emergency Response Plan

    › Use clinical decision-making/critical thinking for emergency response plan.

  » Reporting of Incident/Event/Irregular Occurrence/Variance

    › Evaluate response to error/event/occurrence.

  » Security Plan

    › Use clinical decision making/critical thinking in situations related to security planning.

Overview

- Facility protocols refer to the plans and procedures in place to address specific issues that health care institutions face.
- Nurses must understand their role in relation to the development and implementation of facility protocols.
  - Reporting incidents
  - Disaster planning and emergency response
  - Security plans

REPORTING INCIDENTS

Overview

- Incident reports are records made of unexpected or unusual incidents that affected a client, employee, volunteer, or visitor in a health care facility.
- Incident reports also may be referred to as unusual occurrence or quality variance reports by a health care facility.
- In most states, as long as proper safeguards are employed, incident reports cannot be subpoenaed by clients or used as evidence in lawsuits.
- Examples of circumstances under which an incident report should be filed include the following:
  - Medication errors
  - Procedure/treatment errors
  - Equipment-related injuries/errors
  - Needlestick injuries
  - Client falls/injuries
  - Visitor/volunteer injuries
  - Threat made to client or staff
  - Loss of property (dentures, jewelry, personal wheelchair)
    - Nurses must ensure the safety of clients' valuables. If a client is admitted to the facility and is not accompanied by a family member, the client's valuables should be secured in accordance with facility policy. If an individual requests the client's valuables, the client must identify the person and give that person permission to be in possession of the valuables.

Nursing Role in Reporting Incidents

- In the event of an incident that involves a client, employee, volunteer, or visitor, the nurse's priority is to assess the individual for injuries and institute any immediate care measures necessary to decrease further injury. If it was a client-related incident, the provider should then be notified, and additional tests or treatment should be carried out as prescribed.

- Incident Reports
  - Should be completed by the person who identifies that an unexpected event has occurred. (This may or may not be the individual most directly involved in the incident.)
  - Should be completed as soon as possible and within 24 hr of the incident.
  - Are considered confidential and are not shared with the client. (Nor is it acknowledged to the client that one was completed.)
  - Are not placed in the client's health care record nor mentioned in the client's health care record. However, a description of the incident itself should be documented factually in the client's record.
  - Include an objective description of the incident and actions taken to safeguard the client, as well as assessment and treatment of any injuries sustained.
  - Are forwarded to the risk management department or officer (varies from facility to facility), possibly after being reviewed by the nurse manager.
  - Provide data that may be used in performance improvement studies regarding the incidence of client injuries and care-related errors.

- When completing an incident report, the nurse should include the following:
  - The client's name and hospital number (or visitor's name and address if visitor injury), along with the date, time, and location of the incident
  - A factual description of the incident and injuries incurred, avoiding any assumptions as to the cause of the incident
  - Names of any witnesses to the incident and any client or witness comments regarding the incident
  - Corrective actions that were taken, including notification of the provider and any referrals
  - The name and dose of any medication or identification number of any piece of equipment that was involved in the incident

 View Image: Incident Report

DISASTER PLANNING AND EMERGENCY RESPONSE

Overview

- A disaster is an event that causes serious damage, destruction, injuries, and sometimes death. In many situations, a hospital can manage the event with the support of local resources.

- A mass casualty incident (MCI) is a catastrophic event that overwhelms local resources, and multiple resources (federal and state) are necessary to handle the crisis.

- Each health care facility must have an emergency operating plan (EOP). An essential component of the plan is the provision of training of all personnel regarding each component of the EOP. Nurses should understand their responsibilities in the EOP.

- Health care facilities accredited by the Joint Commission must have an EOP and are mandated to test the plan at least twice a year.

- The EOP should interface with local, state, and federal resources.

- Disasters that health care facilities face include internal and external emergencies.

  ○ Internal emergencies are events that occur within a facility and include loss of electric power or potable water and severe damage or casualties related to fire, severe weather (tornado, hurricane), an explosion, or a terrorist act. Internal emergency readiness includes safety and hazardous materials protocols and infection control policies and practices.

  ○ External emergencies are events that affect a facility indirectly and include severe weather (tornado, hurricane), volcanic eruptions, earthquakes, pandemic flu, chemical plant explosions, industrial accidents, building collapses, major transportation accidents, and terrorist acts (including biological and chemical warfare). External emergency readiness includes a plan for participation in community-wide emergencies and disasters.

- To receive assistance with an MCI, a state must request assistance. Some of the federal programs include the Department of Homeland Security, the National Incident Management System, the National Domestic Preparedness Organization, and the Strategic National Stockpile.

- Nurses should be aware that all health care facilities have color code designations for emergencies. These may vary between institutions, but some examples are:

  ○ Code Red (fire)

  ○ Code Pink (newborn abduction)

  ○ Code Orange (chemical spill)

  ○ Code Blue (mass casualty incident)

  ○ Code Gray (tornado)

- Nurses should be familiar with procedures and policies that outline proper measures to take when one of these emergencies are called.

Nursing Role in Disaster Planning and Emergency Response

- Emergency Response Plans

  ○ Each health care institution must have an emergency preparedness plan that has been developed by a planning committee. This committee reviews information regarding the potential for various types of natural and man-made emergencies depending on the characteristics of the community. Resources necessary to meet the potential emergency also are determined, and a plan is developed that takes into consideration all of these factors.

  ○ Nurses, as well as a cross section of other members of the health care team, should be involved in the development of an EOP for such emergencies. Criteria under which the EOP are activated should be clear. Roles for each employee should be outlined and administrative control determined. A designated area for the area command center should be established, as well as a person to serve as the incident control manager.

  ○ The nurse should create an action plan for personal family needs.

- Mass Casualty Triage
  - Principles of mass casualty triage should be followed in health care institutions involved in a mass casualty event.
  - These differ from the principles of triage that are typically followed during provision of day-to-day services in an emergency or urgent care setting. During mass casualty events, casualties are separated in relation to their potential for survival, and treatment is allocated accordingly. This type of triage is based on doing the greatest good for the greatest number of people.
  - Nurses may find this situation very stressful because clients who are not expected to survive are cared for last.
  - Categories of triage during mass casualty events
    - Emergent category (class I) – Highest priority is given to clients who have life-threatening injuries but also have a high possibility of survival once they are stabilized.
    - Urgent category (class II) – Second-highest priority is given to clients who have major injuries that are not yet life-threatening and usually can wait 45 to 60 min for treatment.
    - Nonurgent category (class III) – The next highest priority is given to clients who have minor injuries that are not life-threatening and do not need immediate attention.
    - Expectant category (class IV) – The lowest priority is given to clients who are not expected to live and will be allowed to die naturally. Comfort measures may be provided, but restorative care will not.
- Discharge/Relocation of Clients
  - During an emergency such as a fire or a mass casualty event, decisions may need to be made regarding discharging clients or relocating them so their beds can be given to clients with higher priority needs.
  - Criteria should be followed when identifying clients who can be safely discharged.
    - Ambulatory clients requiring minimal care should be discharged or relocated first.
    - Clients requiring assistance should be next, and arrangements should made for continuation of their care.
    - Clients who are unstable and/or require nursing care should not be discharged or relocated unless they are in imminent danger.

- Fire
  - If a nurse discovers a fire that threatens the safety of a client, the nurse should use the RACE mnemonic (Rescue, Alarm, Contain, Extinguish) to guide the order of actions.

RACE MNEMONIC	
Rescue	› Rescue the client and other individuals from the area.
Alarm	› Pull the fire alarm, which will activate the EMS response system. › Systems that could increase fire spread are automatically shut down with activation of the alarm.
Contain	› Once the room or area has been cleared, the door leading to the area in which the fire is located as well as the fire doors should be kept closed in order to contain the fire. › Fire doors should be kept closed as much as possible when moving from area to area within the facility to avoid the spread of smoke and fire.
Extinguish	› Make an attempt to extinguish small fires by using a single fire extinguisher, smothering it with a blanket, or dousing it with water (except with an electrical or grease fire). › Complete evacuation of the area should occur if the nurse cannot put the fire out with these methods. › Attempts at extinguishing the fire should only be made when the employee has been properly trained in the safe and proper use of a fire extinguisher and when only one extinguisher is needed.

- Severe Thunderstorm/Tornado
  - Draw shades, and close drapes to protect against shattering glass.
  - Lower all beds to the lowest position, and move beds away from the windows.
  - Place blankets over all clients who are confined to beds.
  - Close all doors.
  - Relocate ambulatory clients into the hallways (away from windows).
  - Do not use elevators.
  - Turn on the severe weather channel to monitor severe weather warnings.
- Biological Incidents
  - Be alert to indications of a possible bioterrorism attack because early detection and management is key.
  - Use appropriate isolation measures.

○ In most instances, infection from biological agents are not spread from one client to another. However, vigilance is of the upmost importance. Management of the incident includes recognition of the occurrence (often the clinical manifestations are similar to other illnesses), directing personnel in the proper use of personal protective equipment, and, in some situations, decontamination and isolation.

INCIDENT	CLINICAL MANIFESTATIONS	TREATMENT/PREVENTION
Inhalational anthrax	› Sore throat › Fever › Cough › Shortness of breath › Muscle aches › Severe dyspnea › Meningitis › Shock	› Oral ciprofloxacin (Cipro) › IV ciprofloxacin › In addition to IV ciprofloxacin, one or two additional antibiotics such as vancomycin, penicillin
Cutaneous anthrax	› Starts as a lesion that may be itchy › Develops into a vesicular lesion that later becomes necrotic with the formation of black eschar › Fever, chills	› Oral ciprofloxacin (Cipro) › Doxycycline (Doryx)
Botulism	› Difficulty swallowing › Double vision › Slurred speech › Descending progressive weakness › Nausea, vomiting, abdominal cramps › Difficulty breathing	› Airway management › Antitoxin › Elimination of toxin
Ebola	› Sore throat › Headache › High temperature › Nausea, vomiting, diarrhea › Internal and external bleeding › Shock	› Treatment: No cure › Supportive care: Minimize invasive procedures › Prevention: Vaccine

INCIDENT	CLINICAL MANIFESTATIONS	TREATMENT/PREVENTION
Plague	› These forms may occur separately or in combination: » Pneumonic plague infects the lungs. The first signs of illness are fever, headache, weakness, and rapidly developing pneumonia with shortness of breath, chest pain, cough, and sometimes bloody or watery sputum. The pneumonia progresses for 2 to 4 days and may cause respiratory failure and shock. » Bubonic plague – swollen, tender lymph glands, fever, headache, chills, and weakness. » Septicemic plague occurs when plague bacteria multiply in the blood. Manifestations include fever, chills, prostration, abdominal pain, shock, and bleeding into skin and other organs.	› Treatment: Early treatment of pneumonic plague is essential. To reduce the chance of death, antibiotics must be given within 24 hr of first symptoms. Streptomycin, gentamicin, the tetracyclines, and chloramphenicol are all effective against pneumonic plague.
Smallpox	› High fever › Fatigue › Severe headache › Rash › Chills › Vomiting › Delirium	› Treatment: No cure › Supportive care: Prevent dehydration, provide skin care, medications for pain and fever › Prevention: Vaccine
Tularemia	› Sudden fever, chills, headache, diarrhea, muscle aches, joint pain, dry cough, progressive weakness › If airborne, life-threatening pneumonia and systemic infection	› Treatment: Streptomycin IV or gentamicin IV or IM are the drugs of choice; in mass causality, use doxycycline or ciprofloxacin. › Prevention: Vaccine under review by the Food and Drug Administration.

- Chemical Incidents
  - Chemical incidents may occur as result of an accident or due to a purposeful action such as terrorism.
  - Take measures to protect self and to avoid contact.
  - Assess and intervene to maintain the client's airway, breathing, and circulation. Administer first aid as needed.

- o Remove the offending chemical by undressing the client and removing all identifiable particulate matter. Provide immediate and prolonged irrigations of contaminated areas. The client's skin should be irrigated with running water with the exception of dry chemicals, such as lye or white phosphorus. In the case of exposure to a dry chemical, brush the agent off of the client's clothing and skin.

  - o Gather a specific history of the injury, if possible (name and concentration of the chemical, duration of exposure).

  - o In the event of a chemical attack, have knowledge of which facilities are open to exposed clients and which are open only to unexposed clients.

  - o Follow the facility's emergency response plans (personal protection measures, handling and disposal of wastes, use of space and equipment, reporting).

- Hazardous Material Incidents

  - o Take measures to protect self and to avoid contact.

  - o Approach the scene with caution.

  - o Identify the hazardous material with available resources (emergency response guidebook, poison control centers). Know the location of the Material Safety Data Sheet (MSDS) manual.

  - o Try to contain the material in one place prior to the arrival of the hazardous materials team.

  - o If individuals are contaminated, decontaminate them as much as possible at the scene or as close as possible to the scene.

    - Don gloves, a gown, a mask, and shoe covers to protect self from contamination.

    - Carefully and slowly remove contaminated clothing so that deposited material does not become airborne.

    - With few exceptions, water is the universal antidote. For biological hazardous materials, wash skin with copious amounts of water and antibacterial soap.

    - Place contaminated materials into large plastic bags, and seal them.

- Radiological Incidents

  - o The amount of exposure is related to the duration of exposure, distance from source, and amount of shielding.

  - o The facility where victims are treated should activate interventions to prevent contamination of treatment areas (floors and furniture should be covered, air vents and ducts should be covered, radiation-contaminated waste should be disposed of according to procedural guidelines).

  - o Staff should wear water-resistant gowns, double-glove, and fully cover their bodies with caps, booties, masks, and goggles.

  - o Staff should wear radiation or dosimetry badges to monitor the amount of their radiation exposure.

  - o Clients initially should be surveyed with a radiation meter to determine amount of contamination.

  - o Decontamination with soap and water and disposable towels should occur prior to the client entering the facility. Water runoff will be contaminated and should be contained.

  - o After decontamination, clients should be resurveyed for residual contamination, and irrigation of the skin should be continued until the client is free of all contamination.

- Bomb Threat
  - When a phone call is received
    - Extend the conversation as long as possible.
    - Listen for distinguishing background noises (music, voices, traffic, airplanes).
    - Note distinguishing voice characteristics of the caller.
    - Ask where and when the bomb is set to explode.
    - Note whether the caller is familiar with the physical arrangement of the facility.
  - If a bomblike device is located, do not touch it. Clear the area, and isolate the device as much as possible by closing doors, for example.
  - Notify the appropriate authorities and personnel (police, administrator, director of nursing).
  - Cooperate with police and others – Assist to conduct search as needed, provide copies of floor plans, have master keys available, and watch for and isolate suspicious objects such as packages and boxes.
  - Keep elevators available for authorities.
  - Remain calm and alert and try not to alarm clients.

SECURITY PLANS

Overview

- All health care facilities should have security plans in place that include preventive, protective, and response measures designed for identified security needs.
- Security issues faced by health care facilities include: admission of potentially dangerous individuals, vandalism, infant abduction, and information theft.
- The International Association for Healthcare Security & Safety (IAHSS) provides recommendations for the development of security plans.

Nursing Role in Security Plans

- Nurses should be aware that security measures include:
  - An identification system that identifies employees, volunteers, physicians, students, and regularly scheduled contract services staff as authorized personnel of the health care facility
  - Electronic security systems in high-risk areas (the maternal newborn unit to prevent infant abductions, the emergency department to prevent unauthorized entrance)
    - Key code access into and out of areas such as the maternal newborn unit
    - Wrist bands that electronically link parents and their infant
    - Alarms integrated with closed-circuit television cameras
- Nurses should be prepared to take immediate action when breaches in security occur. Time is of the essence in preventing a breach in security.

APPLICATION EXERCISES

1. A nurse discovers that a client was administered an antihypertensive medication in error. Number the following actions in the appropriate sequence that the nurse should follow.

_____ A. Call the client's provider.

_____ B. Monitor the client's vital signs.

_____ C. Notify the risk manager.

_____ D. Complete an incident report.

_____ E. Instruct the client to remain in bed until further notice.

2. A nurse manager is explaining the use of incident reports to a group of nurses in an orientation program. Which of the following statements should the nurse manager include? (Select all that apply.)

_____ A. A description of the incident should be documented in the client's health care record.

_____ B. Incident reports should not be shared with the client.

_____ C. Incident reports include a description of the incident and actions taken.

_____ D. A copy of the incident report should be placed in the client's health care record.

_____ E. The risk management department investigates the incident.

3. An individual approaches the door of the maternal newborn unit, states that he is the uncle of a newborn, and asks to be admitted to the unit. Which of the following actions should the nurse take?

A. Admit the individual after he provides the mother's full name and the date and time of the infant's birth.

B. Call security to remove the individual from the area.

C. Instruct the individual to obtain the access code from the family and then return.

D. Call a Code Pink because the man could be attempting to abduct the infant.

4. A community experiences an outbreak of meningitis, and hospital beds are urgently needed. Which of the following clients should the nurse recommend for discharge?

A. 58-year-old man admitted this morning with angina and a history of a coronary artery bypass grafting (CABG) 1 year ago

B. 50-year-old adult with type 2 diabetes mellitus being admitted for rotator cuff surgery

C. 70-year-old adult admitted yesterday with pneumonia and dehydration

D. 65-year-old woman who fell and broke her hip and is scheduled for total hip replacement tomorrow

5. A nurse on a sixth-floor medical surgical unit is advised that a severe weather alert code has been activated. Which of the following actions should the nurse take? (Select all that apply.)

_____ A. Draw window shades and close drapes as protection against shattering glass.

_____ B. Move beds of nonambulatory clients away from windows.

_____ C. Relocate ambulatory clients into the hallways.

_____ D. Use the elevators to move clients to lower levels.

_____ E. Turn the radio on for severe weather warnings.

6. A nurse serving on a disaster preparedness committee is reviewing information about smallpox. Use the ATI Active Learning Template: Systems Disorder to complete this item to include the following:

A. Objective and Subjective Findings: List at least three clinical manifestations.

B. Treatment: List at least two treatment measures.

APPLICATION EXERCISES KEY

1. *Correct order*

    B. Using the nursing process, the first action the nurse should take is to monitor the client for hypotension by monitoring the client's vital signs.

    E. Next, the nurse should instruct the client to remain in bed to prevent a fall due to the risk of hypotension.

    A. Then the nurse should notify the provider, who may prescribe a medication to treat hypotension.

    D. Next, the nurses should complete an incident report that is thorough and accurate.

    C. The last step the nurse should take is to report the incident to the risk manager.

    N NCLEX® Connection: Safety and Infection Control, Reporting of Incident/Event/Irregular Occurrence Variance

2. A. **CORRECT:** The nurse should document a factual description of the event in the client's health care record.

    B. **CORRECT:** Incident reports are confidential and not shared with the client.

    C. **CORRECT:** In addition to providing an accurate description of the event, the nurse also should document the actions taken following the event.

    D. INCORRECT: The incident report is not placed in the client's health care record to shield it from discovery in the event of a lawsuit.

    E. **CORRECT:** Risk managers investigate all incidents as part of the agency's quality assurance program.

    N NCLEX® Connection: Safety and Infection Control, Reporting of Incident/Event/Irregular Occurrence Variance

3. A. INCORRECT: Allowing the individual entrance to the maternal newborn unit could place the infant at risk for abduction. In most instances, this action would not be consistent with facility protocol.

    B. INCORRECT: It is inappropriate to call security because the individual has not displayed threatening behavior.

    C. **CORRECT:** Access codes are provided to clients admitted to the maternal newborn units to protect newborns from abduction and to promote client confidentiality.

    D. INCORRECT: The nurse should not call a Code Pink because the individual has not displayed threatening behavior.

    N NCLEX® Connection: Safety and Infection Control, Security Plan

4. A. INCORRECT: This client is unstable and at risk for a cardiac event. Therefore, he should not be discharged.

   B. **CORRECT:** This client is stable, and he can be safely discharged.

   C. INCORRECT: This client is unstable and is at risk for complications, such as fluid volume deficit, and cannot be safely discharged.

   D. INCORRECT: This client is unstable, and dismissal would place her at risk for further damage to her hip. Therefore, she cannot safety be discharged.

   Ⓝ NCLEX® Connection: Safety and Infection Control, Emergency Response Plan

5. A. **CORRECT:** The nurse should close the window shades and drapes to protect clients from shattering glass.

   B. **CORRECT:** The nurse should move the beds of nonambulatory clients away from windows to protect clients from shattering glass.

   C. **CORRECT:** The nurse should relocate ambulatory clients into the hallway to protect the clients from shattering glass.

   D. INCORRECT: Although it may be safer on a lower floor, it is unsafe to use the elevator.

   E. **CORRECT:** The nurse should use the radio to monitor the activity of the storm.

   Ⓝ NCLEX® Connection: Safety and Infection Control, Emergency Response Plan

6. *Using ATI Active Learning Template: Systems Disorder*

   A. Objective and Subjective Findings
   - High fever
   - Fatigue
   - Severe headache
   - Rash
   - Chills
   - Vomiting
   - Delirium

   B. Treatment
   - Prevent dehydration.
   - Provide skin care.
   - Administer medications for pain and fever.

   Ⓝ NCLEX® Connection: Safety and Infection Control, Emergency Response Plan

REFERENCES

Berman, A. J., & Snyder S. (2012). *Fundamentals of nursing: Concepts, process, and practice* (9th ed.). Upper Saddle River, NJ: Prentice-Hall.

Cherry, B., & Jacob, S. R. (2014). *Contemporary nursing: Issues, trends, & management* (6th ed.). St. Louis, MO: Mosby, Inc.

Marquis, B. L., & Huston, C. J. (2012). *Leadership roles and management functions in nursing: Theory and application* (7th ed.). Philadelphia: Lippincott Williams & Wilkins.

Nies, M., & McEwen, M. (2011). *Community/public health nursing: Promoting the health of populations* (5th ed.). St. Louis, MO: Saunders.

Potter, P. A., Perry, A. G., Stockert, P., & Hall, A. (2013). *Fundamentals of nursing* (8th ed.). St. Louis, MO: Mosby.

Stanhope, M., & Lancaster, J. (2010). *Foundations of nursing in the community* (3nd ed.). St. Louis, MO: Mosby.

Varcarolis, E. M., Carson, V. B., & Shoemaker, N. C. (2010). *Foundations of psychiatric mental health nursing: A clinical approach* (6th ed.). St. Louis, MO: Saunders.

Whitehead, D. K., Weiss, S. A., & Tappen, R. M. (2010). *Essentials of nursing leadership and management* (5th ed.). Philadelphia: F.A. Davis Company.

CONTENT_____ REVIEW MODULE CHAPTER _____

TOPIC DESCRIPTOR_____

Related Content (e.g. delegation, levels of prevention, advance directives)	Underlying Principles	Nursing Interventions › Who? › When? › Why? › How?

Appendix

CONTENT _____ REVIEW MODULE CHAPTER _____

TOPIC DESCRIPTOR_____

DESCRIPTION OF PROCEDURE:

```
                        ┌─────────────────────────────┐
                        │       Procedure Name        │
                        └─────────────────────────────┘
                                      │
        ┌─────────────────────────────┼─────────────────────────────┐
┌───────────────┐           ┌───────────────────┐          ┌─────────────────────┐
│               │           │                   │          │                     │
│  Indications  │           │ Interpretation of │          │ Nursing Interventions│
│               │           │     Findings      │          │  (pre, intra, post) │
│               │           │                   │          │                     │
└───────────────┘           └───────────────────┘          └─────────────────────┘


                        ┌─────────────────────────────┐
                        │   Potential Complications   │
                        └─────────────────────────────┘
                                      │
              ┌───────────────────────┴───────────────────────┐
    ┌───────────────────────┐                      ┌───────────────────────┐
    │                       │                      │                       │
    │ Nursing Interventions │                      │   Client Education    │
    │                       │                      │                       │
    └───────────────────────┘                      └───────────────────────┘
```

Appendix

CONTENT_____ REVIEW MODULE CHAPTER _____

TOPIC DESCRIPTOR_____

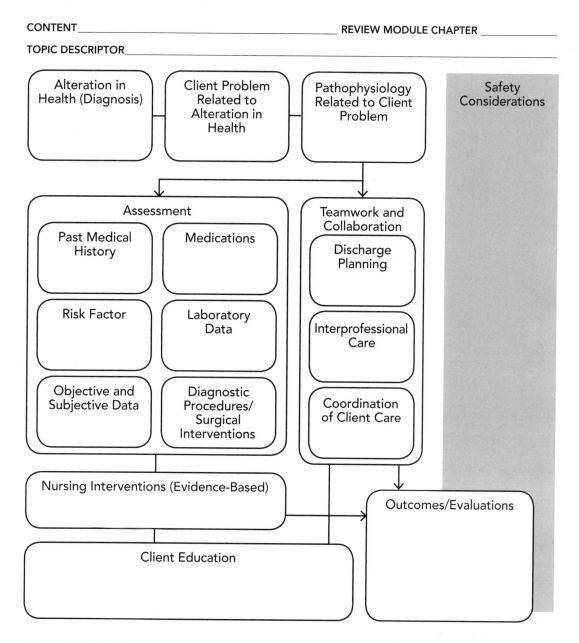

Alteration in Health (Diagnosis)	Client Problem Related to Alteration in Health	Pathophysiology Related to Client Problem	Safety Considerations

Assessment
- Past Medical History
- Medications
- Risk Factor
- Laboratory Data
- Objective and Subjective Data
- Diagnostic Procedures/ Surgical Interventions

Teamwork and Collaboration
- Discharge Planning
- Interprofessional Care
- Coordination of Client Care

Nursing Interventions (Evidence-Based)

Outcomes/Evaluations

Client Education

Appendix

CONTENT _____ REVIEW MODULE CHAPTER _____

TOPIC DESCRIPTOR _____

```
┌─────────────────────────────────────────┐
│          Developmental Stage             │
│                                           │
└─────────────────────────────────────────┘
```

Physical Development	Cognitive Development	Age-Appropriate Activities

```
┌─────────────────────────────────────────┐
│            Health Promotion               │
│                                           │
└─────────────────────────────────────────┘
```

Immunizations	Health Screening	Nutrition	Injury Prevention

Appendix

CONTENT _____ REVIEW MODULE CHAPTER _____

TOPIC DESCRIPTOR_____

MEDICATION _____

EXPECTED PHARMACOLOGICAL ACTION:

Therapeutic Uses

Adverse Effects

Nursing Interventions

Contraindications

Client Education

Medication/Food Interactions

Medication Administration

Evaluation of Medication Effectiveness

Appendix

CONTENT _____ REVIEW MODULE CHAPTER _____

TOPIC DESCRIPTOR_____

DESCRIPTION OF SKILL:

```
                        ┌─────────────────────────────┐
                        │        Procedure Name        │
                        └─────────────────────────────┘
                                       │
        ┌──────────────────────┬───────────────┬──────────────────────┐
┌───────────────┐    ┌──────────────────────┐    ┌──────────────────────┐
│  Indications  │    │ Nursing Interventions│    │  Outcomes/Evaluations │
│               │    │  (pre, intra, post)  │    │                      │
│               │    │                      │    │                      │
└───────────────┘    └──────────────────────┘    └──────────────────────┘

                        ┌─────────────────────────────┐
                        │    Potential Complications    │
                        └─────────────────────────────┘
                                       │
            ┌──────────────────────────┴──────────────────────────┐
    ┌──────────────────────┐                        ┌──────────────────────┐
    │ Nursing Interventions│                        │   Client Education   │
    │                      │                        │                      │
    └──────────────────────┘                        └──────────────────────┘
```

Appendix

CONTENT _____ REVIEW MODULE CHAPTER _____

TOPIC DESCRIPTOR_____

DESCRIPTION OF PROCEDURE:

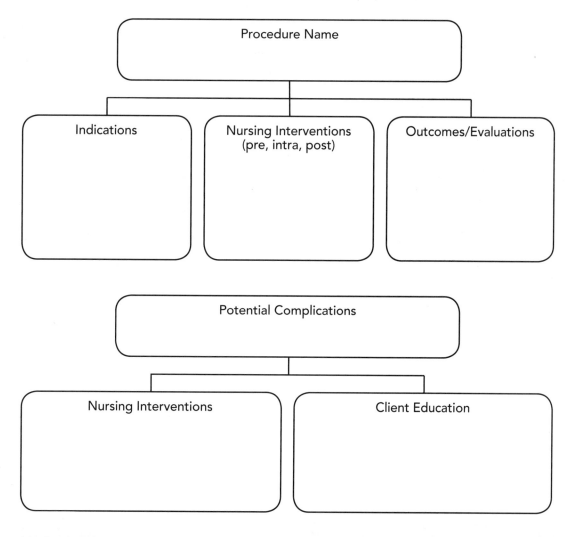